The Comfort of Home™
Multiple Sclerosis Edition

An Illustrated Step-by-Step Guide
for Multiple Sclerosis Caregivers

Other Caregiver Resources from CareTrust Publications:

La Comodidad Del Hogar™ *(Spanish Edition)*
The Comfort of Home™ *Third Edition*
The Comfort of Home™ *Parkison's Disease Edition*
The Comfort of Home™ *Stroke Edition*
The Comfort of Home™ *Caregiving Journal*
The Comfort of Home™ *Caregivers—Let's Take Care of You!* Meditation CD

Newsletters:

The Comfort of Home™ *Caregiver Assistance News*
The Comfort of Home™ *Grand-Parenting News*
The Comfort of Home™ *Caregivers—Let's Take Care of You!*

Visit www.comfortofhome.com

The Comfort of Home™

Multiple Sclerosis Edition

An Illustrated Step-by-Step Guide
for Multiple Sclerosis Caregivers

Maria M. Meyer

and

Paula Derr, RN, BSN, CEN, CCRN

with

Kimberly Koch, MPA and Diane Afes, MA
National Multiple Sclerosis Society

CareTrust Publications LLC
"Caring for you...caring for others."
Portland, Oregon

The Comfort of Home™ Multiple Sclerosis Edition: An Illustrated Step-by-Step Guide for Multiple Sclerosis Caregivers

Published by: CareTrust Publications LLC
P.O. Box 10283
Portland, Oregon 97296-0283
(800) 565-1533
Fax (503) 221-7019

Publisher's Cataloging-in-Publication
(Provided by Quality Books, Inc.)

Meyer, Maria M., 1948-
    The comfort of home. Multiple sclerosis edition : an illustrated
step-by-step guide for multiple sclerosis caregivers /
National Multiple Sclerosis Society ; Maria M. Meyer,
with Paula Derr.
        p. cm.
        Includes index.

        International Standard Book Number ISBN 10: 0-9664767-6-X
        International Standard Book Number ISBN 13: 978-0-9664767-6-7

    1. Home care services—Handbooks, manuals, etc.
2. Caregivers—Handbooks, manuals, etc. 3. Multiple
sclerosis. I. Derr, Paula. II. National Multiple Sclerosis
Society (U.S.) III. Title.

RA645.3.M495 2006   649.8
                QBI06-600168

Cover Art and Text Illustration: Stacey L. Tandberg
Interior Design: Frank Loose
Cover Design: David Kessler
Page Layout: International Graphic Services

Printed in the United States of America.

06 07 08 09 10 / 10 9 8 7 6 5 4 3 2 1

About the Authors

Maria M. Meyer has been a long-time advocate of social causes, beginning with her work as co-founder of the Society for Abused Children of the Children's Home Society of Florida and founding executive director of the Children's Foundation of Greater Miami. When her father-in-law suffered a stroke in 1993, Maria became aware of the need for better information about how to care for an aging parent, a responsibility shared by millions of Americans. That experience led Maria to found CareTrust Publications and to co-author the award-winning guide, *The Comfort of Home™: An Illustrated Step-by-Step Guide for Caregivers*, earning the Benjamin Franklin Award in the health category. She is a keynote speaker and workshop leader on caregiver topics to healthcare professionals and community groups, as well as a Caregiver Community Action Network volunteer for the National Family Caregiver Association.

Paula Derr has been employed by the Sisters of Providence Health System for over 25 years and is clinical educator for three emergency departments in the Portland metropolitan area. She is co-owner of InforMed, which publishes emergency medical services field guides for emergency medical technicians (EMTs), paramedics, firefighters, physicians, and nurses and has co-authored numerous health care articles. For Paula, home care is a family tradition of long standing. For many years, Paula cared for her mother and grandmother in her home while raising two daughters and maintaining her career in nursing and health care management. Her personal and professional experience adds depth to many chapters of this book. Paula is active in several prominent professional organizations—SCCM, ENA, AACN, NFNA—and holds both local and national board positions. Paula is a native Oregonian and lives with her husband in Portland.

The mission of the **National Multiple Sclerosis Society** is to end the devastating effects of multiple sclerosis. The Society and its network of chapters nationwide promote research, educate, advocate on critical issues, and organize a wide range of programs—including support for the newly diagnosed and those living with MS.

If you or someone close to you has recently received a diagnosis of multiple sclerosis, you probably have a lot of questions and concerns. Or, you may be so overwhelmed by the diagnosis that you aren't sure what questions to ask. The National MS Society has developed programs to give you the information and support you need to live comfortably and confidently with this change in your life.

This *Guide* will help you with the questions you may have.

Our Mission

CareTrust Publications is committed to providing high-quality, user-friendly information to those who face an illness or the responsibilities of caring for friends, family, or clients.

❧

Dedication

Because knowledge is empowering, this volume is dedicated to the caregivers and families who live with MS. We hope to add comfort and confidence to their lives.

Dear Caregiver,

Caring for someone with a chronic illness like MS can be deeply satisfying as well as uniquely challenging. Partners, family, and friends can be drawn more closely together when they meet these challenges. Yet, caregiving can also be physically and emotionally exhausting, especially for the person who is the primary caregiver.

The Comfort of Home™ Multiple Sclerosis Edition: An Illustrated Step-by-Step Guide for Multiple Sclerosis Caregivers is a basic but complete guide to answering your questions about caregiving. Although the book discusses issues specific to caring for someone with MS, it also contains valuable information that would be of help to any caregiver. This guide to in-home care uses current best practices in the areas it covers. It offers practical tips for many activities of daily living and the more complicated and stressful situations a caregiver may face. It also includes a wide-ranging list of resources for further reading and study.

The *Guide* is divided into three parts:

Part One, Getting Ready, reviews caregiving options and discusses the financial and legal decisions you may encounter. It shows how to set up a home in a safe and comfortable way for the person whose needs are changing and abilities are declining. Perhaps most important, it teaches you how to communicate better with doctors, nurses, aides, pharmacists and insurance companies to get the services you need.

Part Two, Day by Day, guides you through every aspect of daily care. This may be as basic as bathing or helping someone transfer from a chair to a bed, or as daring as traveling abroad with a person whose health is declining.

Part Three, Additional Resources, provides a list of common medical abbreviations to help you understand the terms that many health care professionals use. There is information about medical specialists who can be part of the health care team and a glossary of terms used to describe and explain symptoms or conditions.

Because a picture is worth a thousand words, we frequently use illustrations throughout the *Guide*. We also include information on organizations and publications that will be invaluable in helping you provide care.

Being a caregiver is not for the timid and fearful. However, having as much knowledge as possible will help you overcome your fears. With this guide in hand, you will understand what help is needed and learn where to find it or how to provide it yourself.

Warm regards,

Maria and Paula

Acknowledgments

The procedures described in this *Guide* are based on research and consultation with experts in the fields of nursing, medicine, accounting, design, and law. The authors thank the innumerable professionals and caregivers who have assisted in the development of this book. We are especially grateful to the following reviewers who made comments on sections of the manuscript during its development. We thank them for their significant contributions, without which the quality and comprehensiveness of this guide would not have been possible.

The National Multiple Sclerosis Society

Kristine S. Beisel
Manager, Special Projects
Client Programs Department

Kathryn K. Dailey, MHA, EdS, MEd
Vice President, Client Programs
    Systems and Resources
Client Programs Department

Linda R. Guiod, RN
Vice President, Chapter Programs
Central New England Chapter

Nancy Holland, RN, EdD
Vice President, Clinical Programs
Research and Clinical Programs
    Department

Rosalind Kalb, PhD
Director, Professional Resource
    Center
Research and Clinical Programs
    Department

Nancy Law
Vice President
Client Programs Department

Dorothy Northrop, MSW
Director, Clinical Programs
Research and Clinical Programs
    Department

Denise Nowack, RD
Executive Vice President
Southern California Chapter

Beverly Noyes, PhD, LPC
Director, Program and Staff
    Development
Client Programs Department

CONTENTS AT A GLANCE

Part Three   *Additional Resources*

CHAPTER

To Our Readers

We believe *The Comfort of Home™ Multiple Sclerosis Edition: An Illustrated Step-by-Step Guide for Multiple Sclerosis Caregivers* reflects currently accepted practice in the areas it covers. However, the authors and publisher assume no liability with respect to the accuracy, completeness, or application of information presented here.

The Comfort of Home™ Multiple Sclerosis Edition is not meant to replace medical care but to add to the medical advice and services you receive from health care professionals. You should seek professional medical advice from a healthcare provider. This book is only a guide; follow your common sense and good judgment.

Neither the authors nor the publisher are engaged in rendering legal, accounting, or other professional advice. Seek the services of a competent professional if legal, architectural, or other expert assistance is required. The guide does not represent Americans with Disabilities Act compliance.

Every effort has been made at the time of publication to provide accurate names, addresses, and phone numbers in the resource sections at the ends of chapters. The resources listed are those that benefit readers nationally. For this reason we have not included many local groups that offer valuable assistance. Failure to include an organization does not mean that it does not provide a valuable service. On the other hand, inclusion does not imply an endorsement. The authors and publisher do not warrant or guarantee any of the products described in this book and did not perform any independent analysis of the products described.

Throughout the book, we use "he" and "she" interchangeably when referring to the caregiver and the person being cared for.

ATTENTION NONPROFIT ORGANIZATIONS, CORPORATIONS, AND PROFESSIONAL ORGANIZATIONS: *The Comfort of Home™ Multiple Sclerosis Edition* is available at special quantity discounts for bulk purchases for gifts, fundraising, or educational training purposes. Special books, book excerpts, or booklets can also be created to fit specific needs. For details, write to CareTrust Publications LLC, P.O. Box 10283, Portland, Oregon 97296-0283, or call 1-800-565-1533.

Part One: Getting Ready

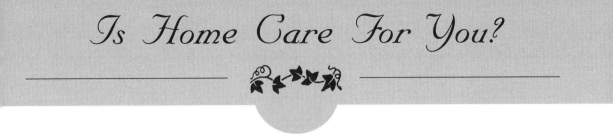

Is Home Care For You?

Is Home Care for You?

*T*he need to provide care for another person arises for many reasons. Often, the person who needs care does not realize it and family members must step in to help make decisions. One of those decisions involves who the caregiver will be and where care will be provided. The choices can be difficult unless you know what to consider.

When one member of the family becomes disabled, roles within the family often change. A person who took care of the family in the past or was the income provider may become dependent, while another person in the family takes on added, often unfamiliar responsibilities. For a single person, the changes may involve a new dependence on non-family members. Just the word "dependence" can cause unpleasant feelings. Being able to talk openly about fears, anxiety, frustration, and doubts can be very helpful in dealing well with these new facts of life.

Discuss chronic care needs with the person's medical team to learn what treatments, adjustments and other changes may be necessary (see chapter 3). For some people, training to provide medical treatments, advice on coping with fatigue and occasional relapses, and some long-range financial planning will be enough. For others, in-home personal assistance is the best option. Sometimes a nursing home or assisted living center is the better choice for everyone involved.

In making the decision for home care, it is important to be realistic about what the person with MS needs, and what you, the caregiver, can provide in terms of time, kinds of care, and financial responsibility. For example, deciding to hire an in-home attendant may be necessary if the primary caregiver works full time. Before this happens, it's important to look at the financial and emotional issues that go along with this decision.

Caregivers need to think about important issues such as independence, privacy, and the financial effect of hiring in-home help. Then the caregiver needs to talk to the person with MS and others living in the home about these issues. How will the family pay for in-home help and how will it find the right person(s) or agency?

Before a person can be hired, the family needs to look at what kind of care is needed: **medical** *(symptom management, occupational or physical therapies, etc.),* **personal care** *(bathing, dressing, using the bathroom, etc.),* **homemaking** *(shopping, errands, laundry, housecleaning), or* **companionship** *(social outlets, safety issues, etc.).*

Your Support System

Sometimes children take on major household and personal care duties when a parent has disability due to MS. While it is positive for children to take on household jobs and tasks, their needs must be carefully balanced with the amount and level of caregiving they are expected to provide. Children are not equipped to handle the stress of being the main or primary caregiver. They should never be in charge of a parent's medical treatments or daily functions such as helping with the bathroom.

Family and friends can help. The first step is to let friends and family know that their help is needed and welcomed. Friends often worry that offering help might seem like meddling, especially when things seem to be going well.

Knowing What Level of Care Is Needed

Before you take on the demanding job of home care, decide what level of care you must provide. Do you need to give:

- minimum assistance?

- moderate assistance?

- maximum assistance?

In order to decide what level of care is needed, you must understand the person's condition and needs in the areas of daily care and health. Generally, these needs fall into two broad groups:

Activities of Daily Living (ADLs) such as eating, bathing, dressing, taking medicine, and going to the toilet.

Instrumental Activities of Daily Living (IADLs) are activities that are important to independence, such as cooking, shopping, housekeeping, getting to the doctor, paying bills, and managing money.

Things to look for in deciding the overall level of care needed are the person's—

- ability to get from bed to wheelchair without help

- ability to move without help in wheelchair or walker

- ability to manage bladder and bowel

- ability to carry out the basic activities of daily living

- ability to call for help

- degree of sight and hearing impairment

- degree of confusion

Also, consider emotional conditions that might require advanced or special levels of care:

- depression

- a need to be with other people or to have privacy

- homesickness

After giving some thought to the level of care that might be needed and the person's condition, abilities, and emotional state, try to place the person you might care for in one of these categories:

Minimum Assistance—This person is basically independent, can handle most household chores and personal care, and needs help with only one or two activities of daily living.

Moderate Assistance—This person needs help with three or more activities of daily living, such as bathing, cooking, or shopping.

Maximum Assistance—This person is unable to care for himself or herself, requires total assistance, and must be placed in a nursing home if no skilled caregiver is available in the home. Care is often provided by professionals, either in the home through home service agencies or in foster care homes, assisted living facilities, or nursing homes. At this level, serious problems are a real possibility.

Deciding Whether Home Care Is Possible

When a person has a chronic condition like multiple sclerosis, daily long-term skilled help with health and personal needs may be in order. Whatever level of care is needed, it can take place in three settings:

- the person's own home
- your home
- residential care facilities, such as a foster care home, assisted living, or a skilled nursing facility

Home Care Considerations

Whether care will take place in your home or in the home of the person who needs care, the following factors must be considered:

- Is there enough room for both the person and items such as a wheelchair, walker, bedside toilet, and lift?
- How accessible is the home if walkers or wheelchairs are used?
- Is a doctor, nurse, or specialist available to supervise care when needed?
- Is there a hospital emergency unit close by?
- Is the home environment safe and supportive and does it allow for some independence?
- Is money available to hire additional help?
- Is the person in question willing to have a caregiver in the home?
- Can the caregiver manage this role along with other family and personal responsibilities?

Things That Must Be Provided

- medication
- meals
- personal care
- housecleaning
- shopping
- transportation
- companionship
- accessibility (wheelchair ramps, support railings, and changes to the bath and shower stall) (See *Preparing the Home,* p. 97)

Benefits of Home Care

- When a caregiver's spouse is supportive, the experience can strengthen the marriage.
- The relationship between the caregiver and the person in care can grow stronger.

- A great deal of money can be saved on health care costs.

Why Home Care May Not Be Possible

- financial reasons (inadequate health insurance to cover the cost of home nursing)
- family limits (lack of time or money)
- the caregiver's lack of physical and emotional strength
- the person's complex medical condition
- the home's physical layout
- the person's desire to live independently of family

Possible Hazards of Home Care

- Possible lack of freedom for the caregiver.
- Caregiver duties may affect the caregiver's job, career, hobbies, and personal life.
- There may be less time for family members, and the caregiver's family relationships may suffer.
- Children in the home may need to be quieter.
- There may be less time for religious services and volunteer work.
- Friends and family may criticize the caregiver's efforts and offer unwelcome advice.
- The caregiver may often be awakened during the night.
- The caregiver may feel unable to control life's events and may suffer from depression, worry, anger, regrets, guilt, and stress.
- Instead of being grateful, the person receiving care may display unpleasant changes in attitude.
- He or she may react to constant daily irritations by lashing out at the caregiver.

- The caregiver may begin to fear the time when he or she may be dependent on someone for care.

- The caregiver may feel obliged to spend personal funds on caregiving.

- The caregiver may become physically ill and emotionally drained.

Outside Help

One of the biggest pitfalls in caregiving is trying to do it all yourself. But other help is available and should be called on whenever possible. That help includes:

- support groups

- day care and respite care, which provide relief for the caregiver

- organizations providing respite care

- pastoral counseling services

- parish nurses

- medical services provided by professionals, such as nurses and therapists

- personal services for the person in your care, such as grooming or dressing, provided by home health aides

- community home health services on a fee basis, such as Visiting Nurse Associations (📖 See *Getting In-Home Help,* p. 45)

Supportive Housing and Care Options

If you believe that home care is not practical for you, many other options exist. Good programs foster independence, dignity, privacy, a very high level of functioning, and connections with the community. However, people who have lived independently all their lives may not be

Checklist **The Ideal Caregiver**

The ideal caregiver is—

✓ *emotionally and physically capable of handling the work*

✓ *able to share duties and responsibilities with other willing family members*

✓ *able to plan solutions and solve problems instead of withdrawing under stress*

✓ *able to speak in a simple and clear way*

✓ *comfortable giving and receiving help*

✓ *trained for the level of care required*

✓ *able to handle unpleasant tasks such as changing diapers, bathing, or cleaning bed sores*

✓ *in good health and has energy, skill, and the ability to adapt*

✓ *able to cope with anger and frustration*

✓ *able to afford respite (back-up) care when necessary*

✓ *able to speak to and understand the care receiver*

✓ *able to make this person feel useful and needed*

✓ *valued by other family members*

✓ *able to adjust to the future needs and wishes of the person in care*

✓ *aware of other care options and willing to explore them*

If you have most of these traits, you may be a good candidate to provide home care. However, consider the list called "Possible Hazards of Home Care" and be honest with yourself about your ability to cope.

suited to live in groups, and those who are mentally alert or are younger may be very unhappy living with people who suffer from dementia.

Keep the above factors in mind when you check out the following:

- **Independent Living Options**—apartment buildings, condos, retirement communities, and single-family homes

- **Semi-independent Living Options**—places that offer the same benefits as independent living but also include meal service and housekeeping as part of the monthly fee, provide help with personal care, keep track of health and medications, and provide special diets. These options are frequently offered in assisted living facilities and group homes.

- **Skilled Care Facilities**—nursing homes

NOTE States use different names for care facilities. The services can also vary, so it is important to check with the facility and each state's licensing agency to confirm exactly which services are offered. For example, in Wyoming, assisted living allows people who are unrelated to share a room. In some other places, living spaces are not shared, except by personal choice.

A Closer Look at the Options

House Sharing—for people who are fully independent

- Two or more unrelated people live together, each with a private bedroom.

- All living areas are shared.

- Chores and expenses are shared.

- Personal-assistant services may be shared.

Group Homes or Adult Foster Care Homes—homes in residential neighborhoods for people whose needs vary, from assistance with individual services to dependent residents with increased nursing services

- Care is given to small groups of people in the primary caregiver's home or with a live-in resident manager/caregiver.

- The home is privately run and provides private or shared rooms with meals, housekeeping, personal care (such as bathing and dressing), keeping track of medication, safety supervision, and some transportation.

- Rates vary according to individual care needs, and Medicaid funding is often available for repayment to those who qualify.

- Staff are qualified and facilities are licensed according to the level of services offered, which can include housekeeping, laundry, personal care assistance, bathing, dressing, grooming, and management of medication and other medical needs, such as injections or inability to control bladder and bowel.

NOTE Some states do not license, inspect, or keep watch over adult foster care homes. Before selecting one, call your local Area Agency on Aging or the state or county Department of Health to see if any complaints have been filed against the home you are considering.

Assisted Living Facilities—for moderate assistance to those who are frail and usually require assistance with activities of daily living

- Each person lives in his or her own apartment.
- An emergency staff is available 24 hours a day.
- Monthly charges are based on the level of service needed.

- Activities such as games, hobbies, crafts, and music are offered.

- Meals, housekeeping, medication management, and nursing assessment are provided.

- Transportation and access to medical services can be arranged.

NOTE There is no national control over these facilities but there is state licensing and regulation. For information on a specific facility, call the ombudsman in your state or the state agency that licenses the facility. (An ombudsman is some-one who looks into complaints made by individuals.)

Continuing Care Retirement Communities—for people who want a range of services from independent living to nursing home care

- These facilities provide a lifetime contract for care.

- They provide or offer meals and can handle special diets.

- They offer housekeeping, scheduled transportation, emergency help, personal care, and activities for fun and learning.

- Many retirement communities require entrance fees that can vary quite a bit.

- They also have monthly fees ranging from several hundred to several thousand dollars.

- Some provide home health care and nursing home care without extra fees.

- Some charge extra for nursing unit residents.

Nursing Homes—for people who require continuous and ongoing nursing assistance or monitoring

Nursing homes typically offer three levels of care:

- **Custodial**—minimal nursing, but help with hygiene, meals, dressing, etc.

- **Intermediate**—help for those who cannot live alone but do not need 24-hour skilled nursing care

- **Skilled Nursing**—intensive 24-hour skilled nursing care

Hospice care is available in all settings as a covered benefit under Medicare. It is also covered for those who receive Medicaid in states that offer hospice coverage under their Medicaid program.

Financing Options

The choice of the right housing option may depend on financing available:

- **Personal Resources** are the most common way to pay.

- **Private Insurance** is helpful, but some policies limit the length and type of benefits and have waiting periods or other limits.

- **Medicare** is for those 65 and older or for people who have been declared disabled by the Social Security Administration. Medicare partially pays for up to 100 days in a skilled nursing care facility after a qualifying related hospitalization of more than three days in a row (not including the day the person leaves the hospital). The financing of hospice care is a separate benefit under Medicare.

- **Medicaid** partially pays for services, including assisted living services in some states, to those who are aged, blind, or have disabilities and have limited financial resources. It is also a major payer for nursing home care.

Checklist **Review Before Deciding on a Facility**

✓ Is a trial period allowed to be sure a person is happy with the facility?

✓ Will the facility refund deposits or entrance fees if the resident dies, chooses to leave, or is asked to leave?

✓ Can a resident choose his or her own apartment? Can personal furniture be used?

✓ Are there younger residents at the facility?

✓ If the person must be away for a short time (even for a hospital stay), will the same apartment be available when he or she returns? Is there a reduced rate during long absences?

✓ If the person marries, can the couple live in the same apartment?

✓ Can the staff handle special diets? Are meal menus posted?

✓ Is transportation provided?

✓ How many people are on staff and how much training have they had?

✓ How often and for what reasons can staff enter the apartment?

✓ Can the resident see his or her own doctor? Who gives out the medications?

✓ Is physical therapy available within the facility?

✓ Is the facility licensed to deal with a resident whose health gets worse or must the person leave if, for example, he or she can no longer walk or begins arguing or fighting with others?

✓ How are decisions made when a person must be moved to another part of the facility?

✓ Is there a 30-day-notice provision for ending the agreement?

✓ Does the facility take Medicare?

✓ Will the facility let a resident "spend down" his or her assets and go on Medicaid?

- **Medigap** policies cover gaps in coverage and may be in place to pay Medicare coinsurance.

(See *Financial Management*, p. 71.)

Points to Review Before Signing a Contract or Lease

Although it is hard to know what problems may arise in a care setting, it is extremely important to take the following steps before signing any legal papers:

- Find out who owns the facility and review the owner's financial status.

- Ask for a copy of the contract and review it with an attorney or financial advisor.

- Do not rely on spoken promises. Make sure the contract is geared to the resident's needs.

- Read the state inspection report on the facility.

- Read all the rules and policies of the facility that are not in the contract.

- Ask to see the facility's license.

Things You Should Know About Facilities

Residents' Rights

General Rights—Residents maintain all their rights guaranteed under the U.S. Constitution, including the right to vote. In addition, they can receive visitors, voice their concerns, form resident councils, and enjoy informed consent, privacy, and freedom of choice.

Privacy—In some cases, a resident may have a roommate. However, residents' rooms are considered private and staff must knock before entering. Also, residents can have private visits with spouses.

Restraints—Only the resident's doctor may order a restraint as part of a care plan and must state the specific restraint's use and period of use. (Use of restraints is strongly discouraged, although not prohibited.)

Lifestyle Choices—Residents do not have as many choices as they would have at home regarding meal times, menu choices, and times for sleep. However, most facilities try to satisfy residents' needs as much as possible.

Ability to Effect Change—Issues can be brought up to the resident council or the long-term-care ombudsman.

Freedom to Leave—A person chooses to enter a facility and has the right to leave at any time regardless of what the family thinks or safety concerns.

NOTE The following describes general guidelines regarding a resident's rights. To obtain specific rules for a particular state, contact the state agency responsible for licensing the facility.

The Resident's Rights When Leaving a Facility

Depending on the admission agreement, a resident must be given written notice 30 days before being moved. If there is a medical emergency, no written notice is required. Generally, a resident may be moved from a facility for the following reasons:

- The person wants to be moved.

- The person must be moved for his or her own good.

- The person must be moved for the good of other residents.

- The facility is not being paid. (However, someone who runs out of money cannot be moved *if* Medicaid will pay.)

- The person came into the facility for special care and that care is completed.

- The facility is being closed.

If the person does not want to leave the facility, IMMEDI-ATELY contact the state agency responsible for licensing the facility and/or Medicaid certification.

If you have questions, call the following:

- the Center for Medicare-Medicaid Services

- the local Senior and Disabled Services Division of the Department of Health and Human Resources

- the long-term-care ombudsman

- the Federal Health Care Financing Administration

- the local Area Agency on Aging

What Family Members and Friends Should Do

- Visit whenever possible.

- Send cards or letters between visits.

- Bring small gifts and treats.

- If allowed, walk around with the person when visiting to provide exercise.

- Listen to the resident's complaints.

- Build a good relationship with the staff.

- Plan off-site outings if appropriate.

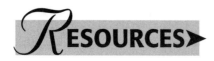

RESOURCES

AARP
601 E Street, NW
Washington, DC 20049
(800) 424-3410
www.aarp.org
Web site provides information on housing and other senior issues.

National Council on Independent Living
1916 Wilson Boulevard, Suite 209
Arlington, VA 22201
(703) 525-3406 (voice)
(703) 525-4153 (tty)
ncil@ncil.org
www.ncil.org
Refers callers to local independent-living centers. Offers publications and advice related to disability issues. Advocates for policy changes.

Assisted Living Facilities and Nursing Homes

American Association of Homes and Services for the Aging
2519 Connecticut Avenue, NW
Washington, DC 20008
(202) 783-2255
(800) 508-9442
www.aahsa.org
Provides information on not-for-profit nursing homes, senior housing facilities, assisted living, and community services. Call for free consumer information brochure.

American Health Care Association/National Center for Assisted Living
1201 L Street, NW
Washington, DC 20005
(202) 842-4444
www.ahca.org
Provides consumer information on services, financing, public policy, nursing facilities, assisted living, and subacute care. Represents more than 10,000 providers of assisted living, nursing care, and subacute care.

Assisted Living Federation of America
11200 Waples Mill Road, Suite 150
Fairfax, VA 22030
(703) 691-8100
www.alfa.org
Offers referrals to local facilities listed by state. Provides free 15-page consumer guide to assisted living.

The Center for Medicare and Medicaid Services has detailed information about the past performance of every Medicare- and Medicaid-certified nursing home in the country. For more information, go to www.medicare.gov, click on Search Tools at the top of the page, and then click on Compare Nursing Homes in Your Area. For a list of **Medicare-certified nursing homes**, call the local office or department on aging.

Respite Services

ARCH National Respite Locator Service
800 Eastowne Drive, Suite 105
Chapel Hill, NC 27514-2204
(919) 490-5577
www.respitelocator.org
Provides caregivers with contact information on respite services in their area.

Eldercare Locator
National Association of Area Agencies on Aging
1730 Rhode Island Avenue, NW, Suite 1200
Washington, DC 20036
(800) 677-1116
www.eldercare.gov
www.aoa.dhhs.gov
Supplies information about many eldercare issues, including respite care. Provides referrals to local respite programs and local Area Agency on Aging.

Books

Creative Caregiving by James Sherman, PhD
Available from National Multiple Sclerosis Society (800) FIGHT-MS (800-344-4867) or www.nationalmssociety.org

Brochures

Brochures designed and published by the National Multiple Sclerosis Society are available at your local chapter. Call (800) FIGHT-MS (800-344-4867) to locate the nearest chapter. Some are available online at www.nationalmssociety.org

A Guide for Caregivers by Tanya Radford

If you don't have access to the Internet, ask your local library to help you locate a Web site.

Using the Health Care Team Effectively

Using the Health Care Team Effectively

*W*hen you care for someone in the home, you must also manage that person's health care. This means choosing a good medical team, keeping costs down, arranging for medical appointments, and getting the best, least expensive medicines. It also means knowing what the insurance rules are and, most important, being an advocate (a supporter) for the person in your care.

Doctors and nurses can focus on physical diagnosis and may ignore the emotional aspects of care. Sometimes they have little time to consider the spiritual aspects of healing. Although you should consult with professionals about the levels of therapy and support needed for the person in your care, you do not have to accept what they suggest or order. Keep asking questions until you completely understand the diagnosis (what is wrong), treatment, and prognosis (likely outcome).

The MS-Specific Health Care Team

MS is a complex condition that can change course quickly and often requires the attention of many specialists. Managing the health of a person with MS involves working with a team of medical specialists who are well-trained in the disease. The person with MS may receive care at an MS center where there are many different kinds of doctors. If not, the caregiver needs to work with the primary-care physician to create such a team and to get all the members to work together. This MS-specific team may include a neurologist (who treats diseases of the nervous system), an MS nurse, a physical therapist, and a neuropsychologist (who studies behavior, the brain, and the nervous system), just to name a few. For a more complete listing of the key members of an MS-specific medical team, refer to the Common Specialists section in Part Three of this book.

It is important for the person with MS not only to have an MS-specific health care team, but also a primary health care team as well for routine, preventive health care, including dental and vision care.

The case manager is another important person of the health care team. Case management is an important resource for families living with MS who are feeling stressed by the demands of the disease and who are unable to handle all the details and red tape of the health and social services network.

Case managers must have a basic understanding of the special needs of a person with MS. Besides assessing needs, a case manager can help come up with a care plan and assist with care decisions and referral to needed services.

Choosing a Doctor

Call your local medical or dental society for the names of doctors who specialize in the field in which you seek care. Think about using doctors who are allied with medical schools. They tend to have the most up-to-date information, especially about complex illnesses like MS.

- Always make sure the doctor is board certified in his or her specialty.

- If the person in your care is enrolled in an HMO, ask if the doctor is planning to change HMOs anytime soon.

- You can contact more than one doctor (for a second opinion). If you are enrolled in Medicare Supplementary Medical Insurance (Part B), Medicare will pay for a second opinion in the same way it pays for other services. After Part B of the deductible has been met, Medicare pays 80 percent of the Medicare-approved amount for a second opinion and will provide the same coverage for a third opinion.

How to Share in Medical Decisions

In the end, medical decision-making is in the hands of the person with MS, the doctor, and the caregiver. Learn to take an active role and become an advocate for yourself and for the person in your care. It has been said that a patient is the senior partner in the patient-doctor relationship. Persons with MS should be encouraged to take charge of their own health care.

Long-Range Considerations

- Find out how the person in your care feels about treatments that prolong life. Respect these views.

- Help the person receiving care to set up an advance directive and power of attorney for health care. (□ See *Planning for the Life Continuum,* p. 85.)

- Share decisions with the doctor and the care receiver and take responsibility for the treatment and its outcomes.

The Doctor–Patient–Caregiver Relationship

- Be aware that doctors must see more patients per day than they once did.

- Be aware that some doctors may have financial reasons for doing too much or too little for those in their care. Specialists are often the only ones with the training needed to treat a serious or chronic condition, so the doctor may refer the person with MS to a specialist.

- If the relationship with the doctor becomes unfriendly, find a new doctor.

- Respect the doctor's time (you may need to have more than one visit to cover all issues).

- If Medicare is the payer, ask if the doctor accepts Medicare assignment. If not, the difference may have to be paid out of pocket.

Preparing for a Visit to the Doctor

- Be prepared to briefly explain the care receiver's and the family's medical history.

- Take a list of questions in order of importance.

- Prepare a list of any MS-related symptoms the person you care for is experiencing.

- Be prepared to ask for written information on the medical situation so you can better understand what the doctor is saying, or bring a small tape recorder.

- You can call the hospital's library or health resource center for help in looking up any questions the doctor does not answer.

NOTE Be sure shots for tetanus, flu, and pneumonia are up-to-date. For those on Medicare, flu and pneumonia shots are covered. Flu shots are recommended for people with MS.

At the Doctor's Office

- Tell the doctor what you hope and expect from the visit and any recommended treatment.

Checklist **Changes to Report to the Doctor**

Contact the doctor **right away** if the following changes occur. Fever may be caused by an infection and should always be reported:

Ability to Move

✓ falls, even if there is no pain

✓ leg pain when walking

✓ painful or limited movement (color of skin over painful areas should be reported)

✓ inability to move

Diet

✓ extreme thirst

✓ lack of thirst

✓ weight loss for no reason

✓ loss of appetite

✓ pain before or after eating

✓ difficulty chewing or swallowing

✓ pain in the gums or teeth

✓ frequent gum infections

Behavior

✓ unusual tiredness or sleepiness

✓ unusual actions (arguing, fighting, anger, or withdrawal)

✓ seeing or hearing things that aren't there (hallucinations)

✓ anxiety

✓ increased confusion

✓ depression

✓ inappropriate or unusual emotions

Bowel/Bladder

✓ bowel movements of an odd color, texture, or amount

✓ feeling faint during bowel movements

✓ vaginal discharge (report color, odor, amount)

✓ draining sores or pain in the penis area

✓ pain when going to the bathroom (unusual color, amount, or odor)

✓ having to go to the bathroom frequently

✓ frequent bladder infections

✓ blood in the urine

✓ pain in the kidney area

Skin

✓ changes in the color of lips, nails, fingers, and toes

✓ odd skin (color, temperature, texture, bruises)

✓ unusual appearance of surgery incisions

✓ sudden skin rashes (bumps, itching)

✓ pressure sores (bedsores)

Bones, Muscles, and Joints

✓ swelling in the arms and legs or around the eyes

✓ twitching or movement that cannot be controlled

✓ tingling or numbness in hands, feet, and other parts of the body

✓ warm, tender joints

✓ redness in the joints

✓ unusual position of arms, legs, fingers, or toes

Chest

✓ chest pain

✓ rapid pulse

✓ problems with breasts (report lumps, discharge, soreness, or draining)

✓ painful breathing (wheezing, shortness of breath)

✓ unusual cough

✓ unusual saliva or mucus (report color and consistency)

Abdomen

✓ stomach pain

✓ vomiting

Head

✓ dizziness

✓ headaches

✓ ear pain, discharge, or change in hearing

✓ eye pain, discharge, redness, blurry vision, or being bothered by light

✓ mouth sores

✓ nose pain (bleeding, bad odor to mucus)

KEEP ASKING QUESTIONS UNTIL YOU ARE SATISFIED. Doctors and other health care professionals have medical know-how, but only you can explain symptoms. Report exactly, in as few words as possible, any unusual symptoms, changes in condition, and complaints the person has.

- If the doctor tells you to do something you know you can't do, such as give medication in the middle of the night, ask if there is another treatment and explain why.

- Insist on talking about the level of care that you believe is appropriate and that agrees with the care receiver's wishes.

- Ask about other options for tests, medications, and surgery.

- Ask why tests or treatments are needed and what the risks are.

- Consider all options, including the pros and cons of "watchful waiting."

- Trust your common sense and if you have doubts, get a second opinion.

Questions to Ask Before Agreeing to Tests, Medications, and Surgery

Before you begin discussing medical treatment with the doctor, explain that the person in your care does not want any unnecessary tests or treatments. Then ask these questions:

- Why is this test needed?

- How long will it take? How soon will the results be in?

- Is the test accurate?

- Is it painful?

- Are there risks with the treatment? Do the benefits outweigh the risks?

- How long will side effects occur and how long will they last?

- Are X-rays really needed?

- Will the doctor review the test report and explain it in detail?

- May a copy of the report be taken home? (If you have questions, ask to talk to the specialist who made the report.)

- If a test is positive, what course of action should be taken?

- Is the condition going to worsen slowly or rapidly?

- What could happen if the person did not have the test?

- How much does the test cost and is there a less costly one?

Questions to Ask the Doctor About Medications

Medications can be costly, confusing to use, and have unwanted side effects. Be sure to ask questions when medicines are prescribed and prescriptions are filled.

- Give the doctor a list of all medications and dosages that the person in your care is now taking, including eye drops, vitamins, and herbal remedies.

- Tell the doctor of any other treatments being used. Sometimes using two or more treatments may be fatal or may keep the new treatment from working.

- Tell the doctor of any allergies or if there are certain foods the person cannot eat (food allergies).

- Understand why each medication is needed and how much it will help the person's condition.

- Ask if pain can be relieved almost completely, and then ask for the medicine that works best.

- Ask how long it takes for the drug to work.

- Find out its side effects.

- Ask if the drug could react with other drugs and what you should do if there are side effects.

- Find out if a change in diet, exercise, reducing stress, or other things can be done.

- If more than one medicine is needed, ask the doctor if they can be taken at the same times each day. If a drug must be taken at a difficult time (for instance, in the middle of the night), ask about another choice.

- Try to find the lowest cost drug. Ask if a generic (non-brand name) drug or another brand in the same drug class is available at a lower cost.

- Be sure that the generic drug will not have a poor effect on the person's condition.

- Ask if a lower dose can be prescribed without bad effects.

- To keep costs down, ask if a higher dose can be safely prescribed and the pill cut in half.

- Ask if you can buy a one-week supply of a new medication to see if the person can handle any possible side effects. Or ask if the physician has free samples to try.

 BUYING MEDICATIONS
Buying medications through mail order is often the cheapest way to buy. Ask if the insurance company has a mail order program.

Questions to Ask the Pharmacist

Some prescription drugs are not covered by health insurance, so shop around for the drug store with the lowest prices, and then stay with it. The pharmacist will come to know the care receiver's condition and can advise you about problems that might come up. Managed care plans are permitted to change doctor's orders by giving you a similar version that is cheaper. Do not try cutting drug costs without talking to you doctor about it first.

- Find out the highest allowable charge for a particular drug.

- Ask what over-the-counter drugs the pharmacist suggests for the person's condition (it may be necessary to take more of the drug if it is over-the-counter).

- Ask if the insurance company will pay for the drug the doctor prescribed.

- Ask if the doctor will be called to approve the switch to another drug.

- Find out what generic drug can be used instead of the prescription drug.

- Ask if the generic drug can cause side effects and when the doctor should be called about them.

- Ask if using more than one drug can cause unsafe drug interactions.

- Ask if the pharmacy's computer will alert the pharmacist about drug-interactions or side effects before the prescription is filled.

- Find out the risks of not taking the medicine.

- Find out the risks of not finishing the prescription.

- If you are caring for someone who will be taking several medications on his or her own, find a drug store that has easy-to-use packaging.

- Ask if the medicine can be put in a large easy-to-open container with a label in large print.

- Ask if an overdose of the medicine is dangerous.

- Ask if the person can drink alcohol or smoke while taking the medication.

- Ask if the medicine must be taken with a meal, with water or milk, etc.
- When the person needs many expensive drugs, find out if you can get a discount or work out a payment plan.

> *Tip* **MEDICAL ALERT**
> A person with MS may want to wear a medical alert bracelet, or carry a card, that lists the medications he or she is currently taking.

Questions to Ask About Surgery

Surgery is a serious step. Ask as many questions as you need before deciding to go ahead.

- Why does the person need the surgery?
- Will the surgery stop the problem or merely slow it down?
- What are the other choices?
- Can it be done on an outpatient basis?
- What will happen if surgery is not done?
- Where will the surgery be done? When?
- Is there a less expensive hospital?
- Will the surgeon you spoke to do the surgery or will it be assigned to another doctor? (When going into surgery, put the surgeon's name on the release form to ensure that the named surgeon is the one who does the operation.)
- How many surgeries of this type has the doctor performed? (Generally, the more times the surgeon has

performed an operation, the higher the success rate will be.)

- What is the doctor's success rate with this type of surgery?

- What are the anesthesiologist's qualifications?

- What can go wrong?

- How much will the surgery cost, and is it covered by insurance?

- What other specialists can I ask for a second opinion? (Medicaid and Medicare usually pay for second opinions. Doctors expect people to get a second opinion when surgery is needed, and they should help you get one.)

MEDICAL RECORDS

To save costs, have all medical records and tests sent to the second doctor. Also, if possible, bring the important ones with you.

Even the experts can disagree about the best treatment. The final decision is yours.

Alternative Treatments

A healthy lifestyle is encouraged by most medical providers. Use caution if you decide to try a different kind of treatment (known as complementary or alternative treatment). There are many claims of "cures" for people with MS that cannot be proved. Look before you leap and follow these commonsense guidelines:

- Be on guard against anyone who says to stop seeing a conventional (regular) doctor or to stop taking pre-scribed medicine.

- Look into the background of any treatment provider.

- Discuss the alternative or complementary therapy with your doctor.

- Figure out the costs of the treatments.

- Do not abandon conventional therapy.

- Keep a written account of the experience.

Mental Health Treatment

Strong emotions are a normal part of long-term illness. Counseling and support groups are a very helpful way of dealing with these feelings.

- For one who is depressed and needs therapy, ask the primary care doctor to give you the name of a therapist.

- Be aware that many people are embarrassed about mental health problems and may not want to seek care.

Dental Care

Dental care is important for overall wellness. For low-cost dental programs, check with university dental schools or the local Area Agency on Aging.

- Tell the dentist all the medications the person is taking before starting dental treatment.

- Try to go to a dentist who is familiar with the person's disease. (Ask your local National MS Society chapter or support group for a list of names.)

- Find out how many visits will be needed each year.

- Ask if the office and dental chair are accessible, if that is needed.

- Ask about low-cost options to the treatment the dentist suggests.

- Ask if X-rays are really necessary.

- Find out the cost of dentures, but don't trust prices that seem too good to be true. Cheap dentures may not fit correctly.

- When seeking another opinion, have all medical records and tests sent to the second dentist.

Vision Care

Regular eye exams every two years by a specialist in eye disease (ophthalmologist) or someone who examines the eyes (optometrist) are necessary. These exams can also spot or detect other serious diseases such as diabetes. Finding and treating disease early can prevent serious diseases from getting worse and leading to blindness.

- Tell the doctor of any medicines the person is taking.

- Tell the doctor if there is a family history of glaucoma.

- Get a yearly eye exam for a person with diabetes.

- Contact your state's Commission for the Blind for information on self-help organizations for those with low vision.

- Ask for help in finding products ("talking" watches, etc.) and aids that will help the person adjust to low vision.

- Seek out radio stations that have programs of newspaper readings.

Eye problems can occur frequently in MS, but rarely result in total loss or blindness. Blindness that lasts for a brief period may occur at the time of an acute flare-up. It is often due to an inflamed optic nerve, called optic neuritis, and usually clears in 4 to 12 weeks.

Other visual problems in MS may result in "jumping vision" (eye movements that cannot be controlled, called nystagmus). Double vision also occurs commonly in MS. It may go away on its own.

NOTE Danger signs to watch for are changes in the color or size of an object when one eye is covered or when straight poles appear bent or wavy. See an ophthalmologist (eye doctor) without delay.

How to Watch Out for Someone's Best Interests in the Hospital

A person in the hospital is at greater risk than others, so be ready to keep tabs on treatments, ask questions, and act as an advocate.

- If the Patients' Bill of Rights is not posted in a place where it can be seen, ask for a copy.

- Agree only to treatments that have been thoroughly explained.

- If something is not being done and you think it should be, ask why.

- Be friendly and show respect to hospital staff. They will probably respond better to you and to the person in your care. Bad feelings between family members and staff may cause the staff to avoid the person.

- Assist with the person's grooming and care.

- Speak up if you notice doctors or nurses examining anyone without first washing their hands.

- Check all bills and ask questions about anything that isn't clear to you.

NOTE According to federal law, a hospital must release patients in a *safe manner* or else must keep them in the hospital. Letting a patient leave the hospital is not wise if the person has constant fever, infection or pain that cannot be controlled, confusion, disorientation (no sense of time or place), or is unable to take food and liquids by mouth. However, in some cases, it may be better for the person to be released because the noise and risk of catching other diseases may make it more difficult to recover. If you plan to appeal a discharge, understand the rules of Medicare, Medicaid, the HMO, or insurance plan.

When You Doubt the Time Is Right for Discharge

- State your doubts in a simple letter to the hospital's director or the health plan's medical director. (Rules vary from state to state.)

- Meet with the hospital's discharge planner.

- Ask if the hospital is following the usual policy for the condition.

- Explain any special reasons that make you think it is unwise to discharge the person.

- Ask if the hospital rules can be changed to cover this special case.

- Remember that anyone has the right to appeal a discharge.

- Get your doctor's help in the appeal, but understand that he or she may have different reasons for wanting to discharge the person.

Checklist **Coming Home from the Hospital**

✓ Assess the person's condition and needs.

✓ Understand the diagnosis (what is wrong) and prognosis (what will happen).

✓ Become part of the health care team (doctor, nurse, therapists) so you can learn how to provide care.

✓ Get complete written instructions from the doctor. If there is anything you don't understand, ASK QUESTIONS.

✓ Arrange follow-up care from the doctor.

✓ Develop a plan of care with the doctor. (📖 See **Setting up a Plan of Care,** p. 141.)

✓ Meet with the hospital's social worker or discharge planner to determine home care benefits.

✓ Understand in-home assistance options. (📖 See **Getting In-Home Help,** p. 45.)

✓ Arrange for in-home help.

✓ Arrange physical, occupational, and speech therapy as needed.

✓ Find out if medicine is provided by the hospital to take home. If not, you will have to have prescriptions filled before you take the person home.

✓ Prepare the home. (📖 See **Preparing the Home,** p. 97.)

✓ Buy needed supplies; rent, borrow, or buy equipment such as wheelchairs, crutches, and walkers.

✓ Take home all personal items.

✓ Check with the hospital cashier for discharge payment requirements.

✓ Arrange transportation (an ambulance or van if your car will not do).

NOTE Do not hesitate to call the hospital staff member (ombudsman) who is responsible for patients' rights.

Case Management

Case management is an important resource for families living with MS. It is easy to become stressed out with the demands of the disease and with the red tape of the health care and social services network. Case managers need to have a basic understanding of the special needs of persons with MS.

Case management skills are very helpful to families when there is a change in the person's physical state or in awareness and understanding. Should this happen, a case manager can take another look at the person's needs and at community supports. This may be necessary in the following instances:

- when the person loses the ability to process information and help is needed to identify issues and provide follow-up with a course of action

- when there is a change in the caregiver situation or support network that can easily become a crisis for the family as a whole

- when there are fewer financial resources and the family is no longer able to pay for the resources they need

- when safety issues arise that can put the person with MS at greater risk

These issues and others require that case management continue as a long-term resource so that the case manager can step in when needed to provide more support.
To learn more about case management or find a case manager in your area, contact:

- your local chapter of the National Multiple Sclerosis Society at (800) FIGHT-MS (800-344-4867)

- the National Association of Professional Geriatric Care Managers, Inc. at (520) 881-8008 or www.findacare manager.org

- your local Visiting Nurse Association

- Area Office on Aging

- hospital discharge planners

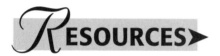

RESOURCES

For free or low-cost resources, contact local consumer health resource and information centers (check the local hospital system or phone book) and local health agencies or associations (American Heart Association, American Diabetes Association, National Multiple Sclerosis Society, and others). In addition, local chapters of the National MS Society maintain a database of health care providers in your area. It is important to have a general wellness health-care team as well as the MS-specific team.

Doctor's Guide to the Internet—Patient Edition
www.pslgroup.com/PTGUIDE.HTM
Provides information for specific diseases and gives pointers to other Internet sites of medical information.

Go Ask Alice!
www.goaskalice.columbia.edu/about.html
Provides helpful information and lets you post health-related questions.

The Health Resource, Inc.
933 Faulkner Street
Conway, AR 72034
(800) 949-0090; (501) 329-5272; Fax (501) 329-9489
www.thehealthresource.com
Provides clients with personalized detailed reports on their specific medical conditions. These reports contain conventional and alternative treatments and information on current research, nutrition, self-help measures, specialists, and resource organizations. Reports on any non-cancer condition are $295, or $395 for complex issues, and contain 50 to 100 pages. Reports on any cancer condition are $395 and contain 150 to 200 pages. Shipping is additional.

National Multiple Sclerosis Society
(800) FIGHT-MS (800-344-4867)
www.nationalmssociety.org

Rocky Mountain MS Center
www.ms-cam.org

University of Washington
www.uwmedicine.org
A great storehouse of general health information on all topics.

Information About Eyesight

Lighthouse International
111 E. 59th Street
New York, NY 10022
(800) 829-0500
www.lighthouse.org

Lions Club International
300 W. 22nd Street
Oak Brook, IL 60523
www.lionsclub.org
(630) 571-5466

National Association for Visually Handicapped
22 West 21st Street, 6th floor
New York, NY 10010
(212) 889-3141
www.navh.org

National Federation of the Blind
1800 Johnson Street
Baltimore, MD 21230
(410) 659-9314
www.nfb.org

Publications

Clear Thinking About Alternative Therapies, available from National Multiple Sclerosis Society (800) FIGHT-MS (800-344-4867) or www.nationalmssociety.org

Choosing the Right Health Care Provider, available from National Multiple Sclerosis Society (800) FIGHT-MS (800-344-4867) or www.nationalmssociety.org

Also available from the National Multiple Sclerosis Society:

Dental Health: The Basic Facts.
Preventative Care Recommended for Adults with MS: The Basic Facts.
Vision Problems: Basic Facts.

A Family Caregiver's Guide to Hospital Discharge Planning, a publication of the National Alliance for Caregiving and the United Hospital Fund of New York. Available at www.caregiving.org

If you don't have access to the Internet, ask your local library to help you locate a Web site.

Getting In-Home Help

Getting In-Home Help

*G*etting help with caregiving in the home involves the following options:

- *Using a home health care agency (typical fee range: $50 to $150 per visit through a private agency)*

- *Hiring someone privately (typical fee range: $12 to $15 per hour; the cost of assistance is based on the category of professional or his or her experience)*

- *Performing all caregiving duties with the assistance of family and friends.*

Use a Home Health Care Agency

Home Health Care Agencies are for-profit, nonprofit, or are run by the government. They provide personal care, skilled care, instructions for caregiver and care receiver, and supervision. They usually provide certified nurse assistants (CNAs), sometimes called home health aides; registered nurses (RNs); licensed practical nurses (LPNs); physical therapists, occupational therapists, and speech therapists. (A doctor's order is required in order to get coverage for skilled-care nursing in the home.) These agencies help plan services and care that match the health, social, and financial needs of the client.

Definitions for Agencies

There are a number of terms to describe an agency's services and how it is able to do what it does. Study the terms carefully before looking into the agencies in your area.

Accredited—Services have been reviewed by a nonprofit organization interested in quality home health care.

Bonded—The agency has paid a fixed dollar amount in order to be bonded. In the event of a court action the bond pays the penalties. (Being bonded does not ensure good service.)

Certified—The agency has met the lowest federal standards for care and takes part in the Medicare program.

Certified Health Personnel—Those who work for the agency meet the standards of a licensing agency for the state.

Insurance Claims Honored—The agency will look into insurance benefits and will accept assignment of benefits (meaning the insurance company pays the agency directly).

Licensed—The agency has met the requirements to run its business (in those states that oversee home health care agencies).

Licensed Health Personnel—The personnel (staff) of the agency have passed the state licensing exam for that profession.

Screened—References have been checked; a criminal background check may or may not have been made.

How to Pay for Using an Agency

Paying for care from an agency ranges from Medicare to private pay to long-term-care insurance to state and county programs.

Medicare

To be eligible for the Medicare home-health benefit, a person must be basically unable to leave the house (homebound) and need skilled care.

- Medicare pays the full cost of medically necessary home health visits by a Medicare-approved home health agency.

- Medicare and most insurers will pay for skilled care (such as a registered nurse) that is not for maintenance.

- The person must be as unable to care for himself or herself as someone who would be in a nursing home.

 State rules vary on who is eligible, so check with your area Medicare office for local rules.

State and County Personal Assistance Programs

- The person receiving services may need to be certified as eligible for a nursing home.

- Many programs require that the person be at a low-income level.

- Funding may come from Medicaid waivers and funding is sometimes not regular.

Private Pay

- If a person does not qualify for public funds, he or she must pay with long-term-care insurance or pay privately.

- Care management through Area Agencies on Aging may be free or offered on a sliding scale, based on a person's income.

What the Home Health Care Agency Will Do

- carry out an in-home visit

- look into insurance benefits and publicly funded benefits

- ask for an assignment of benefits (where payments are made by the insurer directly to the agency)

- ask you to sign a form to release medical information

- ask you to agree to and sign a service contract

- carry out an assessment (by the director of nurses) to determine the level of care required

- discuss the costs of suggested services

- come up with a plan of care that shows the person's diagnosis (what is wrong), functional limitations (what the person can and cannot do), medications, special diet, what services are provided by agency, advice for care, and list of equipment needed

- give you a written copy of the plan of care

- send a copy of the plan of care to the person's doctor

- select and send the right caregivers, only to the level of care needed, to the person's home

- adjust services to meet changing needs

Expect the Agency to:

- be an advocate, advisor, and service planner and to share information clearly with you

- give a full professional assessment

- get in touch with the care receiver's doctor as part of the assessment process

- have knowledge of long-term-care services and how to pay for them

- fill out the paperwork for publicly funded benefits

- show no bias or favor to service providers who may have contracts with the agency

- provide confidential treatment that will not be talked about with others

Checklist **Things to Do Before Selecting an Agency**

✓ Interview several agencies.

✓ Get references and CHECK THEM.

✓ Make a list of services you want and ask the agency what it will cost.

✓ Ask what the steps are in the care planning and management process and how long each will take.

✓ Find out how and when you can contact the care manager.

✓ Find out if the agency has a system for sending a substitute (stand-in) aide if the regular one doesn't show up.

✓ Ask if the agency will replace the aide if that aide and the person in care do not get along.

✓ Ask about the skills and ongoing training of personnel.

✓ Ask how they keep track of the quality of services.

✓ Ask for the services needed by the person in care, even if the insurance company is trying to hold down costs.

✓ Be aware that if a social service agency is providing the care services, they may limit you to only the services that they provide.

✓ Ask them to tell you about any referral-fee agreements they may have with nursing homes or other care facilities.

✓ Know what you have to do to lodge complaints against the agency with the state ombudsman or long-term-care office.

✓ Get in touch with the local/state Division for Aging Services to check for complaints against a particular agency.

- provide a written account of care when you ask for it
- have a proven track record of being honest, reliable, and trusted if the agency handles a person's money

Hire Someone Privately—A Personal Assistant

Even if you decide not to use an agency, a health care professional can help you decide how to prepare the home. They can give advice about needed supplies and where to purchase them and set up a care program. However, when you hire someone privately, you must assume payroll responsibility, complete required government forms (such as Social Security), decide on fringe benefits, track travel expenses, and provide a detailed list of tasks to be done.

Tip

WHEN YOU START CALLING FOR RESOURCES:

- Have information ready, such as what services will be needed and personal information, such as the age of the person, date of birth, social security number, etc.).
- Have your questions written down and ready.
- Realize that to be eligible for some services there may be income, age, or geographic requirements.
- COMMUNICATE, COMMUNICATE, COMMUNICATE what you want and need!

Where to Find Help

- Yellow Pages under Nurses, Nursing Services, Social Service Organizations, Home Health Services, and Senior Services
- commercial agencies, which operate like temp employment agencies, screen applicants, and provide you with a list of candidates

- nonprofit agencies, such as the Visiting Nurse Association, which may charge a fee on a sliding scale (based on ability to pay)

- public health nursing through a county social service department (if you have no insurance or money)

- hospital discharge planner

- hospital-based home health agencies

- the school of nursing at a local community college

- college employment offices

- hospices (call the National Hospice Organization)

- nurses' registries

- Catholic Charities, Jewish Family Services, and other faith-based groups

- the American Red Cross

- churches, synagogues, mosques

- a nearby nursing home employee who seeks part-time work

- an adult relative whom you would pay a fair hourly wage for services

Types of Health Care Professionals

Registered Nurse (RN)—has at least 2 years of school training and is licensed by the state Board of Nursing Examiners

Licensed Practical Nurse (LPN)—has finished a one-year course of study and is licensed by the state Board of Licensed Vocational Nurses

Certified Nurses Aide (CNA)—has finished 70 hours of classes and 50 hours of clinical practice in a nursing center setting; must pass a test and register with the State Board of Nursing

Home Health Aide—is screened on the basis of work experience; training and requirements differ from state to state

Someone who is taking classes or is in a training program that leads to one of the above professions might be able to help with care.

Tax Rules You Must Follow If You Hire Privately

- If you paid more than $1,400 in 2005 or $1,500 in 2006, you are required to pay Medicare and Social Security tax.

- You may use federal income tax return Form 1040 to pay the Social Security, Medicare, and Federal Unemployment (FUTA) taxes. Ask the Internal Revenue Service for the *Household Employer's Tax Guide*.

- For tax information, call the Social Security office. Look in the front of your phone book under State Government.

How to Screen a Personal Hire

- Check licenses, training, experience, and references.
- Be sure the person who is applying for hire has malpractice or liability insurance.
- Run a criminal background check and a driving record check (through a private investigator). Also, ask to see the person's insurance card.
- Find out if the person has a special skill (for example, working with care receivers who have multiple sclerosis or other neurological disorders).
- Decide whether the person is someone who can meet the emotional needs of the person in your care.
- Consider his or her personal habits.
- Find out if he or she is a smoker or nonsmoker.

You can hire a private investigator to look at public records and check on education and licenses, driving history, and previous employers. This service can be obtained anywhere in the country.

Questions to Ask of the Applicant's References:

When someone is going to be hired, ask for the names of people who can tell you about this person's work and personal habits. Here are some questions you can ask:

- How long have you known this person?
- Did this person work for you?
- Is this person reliable, on time for work, patient, able to adjust as things change, able to be trusted, and polite?
- How does this person handle disagreements and emergencies?
- How well does this person follow directions, respond to requests, and take advice?

Perform All Caregiving Duties Yourself

If you decide to provide all the caregiving yourself, you can receive training at the following places:

- social service agencies
- hospitals
- community schools
- the American Red Cross

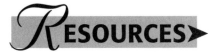
RESOURCES ➤

Family Caregiver Alliance
690 Market Street, Suite 600
San Francisco, CA 94104
(800) 445-8106; 415-434-3388 Fax: (415) 434-3508
www.caregiver.org
E-mail: info@caregiver.org
Resource center for caregivers of people with chronic disabling conditions. The Web site provides information on services and programs in education, research, and advocacy.

National Family Caregivers Association
10400 Connecticut Avenue, Suite 500
Kensington, MD 20895-3944
(800) 896-3650; (301) 942-6430
www.thefamilycaregiver.org
Email: info@thefamilycaregiver.org
The Association supports, empowers, educates, and speaks up for more than 50 million Americans who care for a chronically ill, aged, or disabled person.

National Multiple Sclerosis Society
(800) FIGHT-MS (800-344-4867)
www.nationalmssociety.org

Home Care Agencies/Hiring Help

The Center for Applied Gerontology, Council for Jewish Elderly
3003 W. Touhy Avenue
Chicago, IL 60645.
(773) 508-1000
E-mail: cag@cje.net
www.cje.net/professional/cag_orderform_2.pdf
Offers a 32-page pamphlet "Someone Who Cares: A Guide to Hiring an In-Home Caregiver." $9.95 plus $3.50 shipping and handling.

National Association for Home Care
228 Seventh Street, SE
Washington, DC 20003
(202) 547-7424
www.nahc.org
Provides referrals to state associations, which can refer callers to local agencies. Offers publications, including the free pamphlet "How to Choose a Home Care Agency: A Consumer's Guide." Information on finding help, interviewing, reference checking, training, being a good manager, maintaining a good working and personal relationship, problems that might arise and how best to solve them, service dogs, assistive technology, and tax responsibilities. Contains sample forms and letters.

Publications

Avoiding Attendants from Hell: A Practical Guide to Finding, Hiring and Keeping Personal Care Attendants by June Price

Hiring Help at Home: The Basic Facts (MS Basic Facts Series) published by the National Multiple Sclerosis Society. To request a copy call (800) FIGHT-MS (800-344-4867).

Managing Personal Assistants: A Consumer Guide, published by Paralyzed Veterans of America. To purchase a copy call (888) 860-7244, or download online at www.pva.org/cgi-bin/pvastore/products.cgi?id=2

If you don't have access to the Internet, ask your local library to help you locate a Web site.

Paying for Care

Paying for Care

$\mathcal{Y}$ou can look to many sources for help in paying for care. Some are public, while others are private or volunteer. The most common ways to pay for home care are as follows:

- personal and family resources

- private insurance

- Medicare, Medicaid, Department of Veterans Affairs, and Title programs

- community-based services

Assessment of Financial Resources

First, complete a personal financial resources assessment by doing the following steps:

- Look at current assets, where your income comes from, and insurance entitlements.

- Prepare a budget and figure out what your future income might be from all sources.

- Confirm the qualifications, retirement benefits, and Social Security status of the person in your care.

- Figure as closely as possible the expenses of professional care and equipment. Include any medical procedures likely to be needed.

- Check on the person's personal tax status and find out what care items and expenses are deductible.

- Find out if the person's health insurance or employer's workers' compensation policy has home health care benefits.

- Figure out how much money the person will need.

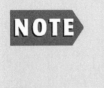

NOTE Think about making the person in your care a "dependent" and thus be able to transfer medical expenses to a taxpayer who can make use of medical deductions. (📖 See *Financial Management and Tax Planning*, p. 71.)

Public Pay Programs

Medicare

Medicare is a federal health insurance program. It provides health care benefits to all Americans 65 and older and to those who have been determined to be "disabled" according to the Social Security Administration. There are constant changes in Medicare policies, requirements, and forms. Therefore, it is always best to get the most current information on benefits by calling the Medicare Hotline (p. 68) or your hospital's social worker.

Things That Affect Medicare Eligibility

Whether the Person Is Homebound—Medicare will pay for certain home health care services only if the person is confined to the home and requires part-time skilled (nursing) services or therapy. Medicare does not cover ongoing custodial (maintenance) care. "Confined to home" does not mean bedridden. It means that a person cannot leave home except for medical care and requires help to get there. (Brief absences from the home do not affect eligibility.)

In order for treatments, services, and supplies to be paid, they must be ordered by a doctor. They must also be provided by a home health agency certified by Medicare and the state health department.

Whether Care Is Intermittent (periodic)—In order to be covered, skilled services are required. Medicare is not designed to meet chronic ongoing needs that are considered "custodial" rather than "skilled."

Medicare Generally Pays for the Following:

- almost all costs of skilled care, such as doctors, nurses, and specialists
- various types of therapy—occupational, physical, speech-language
- home health services
- medical supplies and equipment
- personal care by home health aides (such as bathing, dressing, fixing meals, even light housekeeping and counseling) after discharge from a hospital or nursing home

Medicare Part D

Beginning January 1, 2006, Medicare will cover prescription drugs. There are two basic ways to sign up for this coverage. If you have traditional Medicare (Part A for hospital services and Part B for doctor and outpatient health-care providers), you may sign up for a stand-alone Medicare Part D prescription drug plan. You can also choose a managed care plan under Medicare Advantage. These plans restrict you to only the doctors on the managed-care provider's list. They also have a prescription drug plan. All plans are from private companies that have been approved by Medicare.

Help is available to pay for copayments and premiums for those whose incomes are low enough to be eligible. A person must apply to the Social Security Administration for financial assistance.

> **NOTE** Phrases like "intermittent care," "skilled care," and "homebound" are not precisely defined. They are different from region to region, and the type and availability of coverage by Medicare may be different as well.

Services NOT covered by Medicare

Full-time nursing care at home, drugs, meals delivered to the home, homemaker chore services *not* related to care, and personal care services are usually not covered by Medicare. (📖 See *Hospice Care*, p. 88.)

> **NOTE** A caregiver who has power of attorney for a person on Medicare (the beneficiary) must send written permission to the person's Medicare Part B carrier. Send a letter with the person's name, number, signature, and a statement that the caregiver can act on behalf of the beneficiary. The form must list start and end dates.
>
> If there is a dispute about a repayment from Medicare, a review may be requested by filing a claim with the Medicare carrier.

Medicare Part B Insurance

Medicare Part B insurance costs $88.50 per month (as of 2006) and offers extra benefits to basic Medicare coverage. It pays for tests, doctor's office visits, lab services, and home health care. A $100 deductible applies.

Medicare Supplemental Insurance (Medigap)

To pay for benefits not covered by Medicare, this private health insurance option is available. It pays for noncovered services only—for example, hospital deductibles, doctor copayments, and eyeglasses—but does not cover long-term care services. Coverage depends on the plan you buy.

For anyone who has Medicare HMO coverage, Medigap insurance may not be necessary because those individuals only make a small copayment but do not pay a deductible for doctor's visits.

> **NOTE** It is illegal for an insurance company or agent to sell you a second Medigap policy unless you put in writing that you intend to end the Medigap policy you have. The federal toll-free telephone number for filing complaints is (800) 638-6833.

Medicaid

Medicaid pays for the medical care of low-income elderly persons or those whose assets have been used up while paying for their own care. Eligibility depends on monthly income limits and personal assets. Coverage includes nursing facilities, assisted living, foster care, and certain types of home care. Each state runs its own Medicaid program, and so eligibility and coverage can vary. Some states have set up Medicaid Waiver programs, which pay for home and community-based services that would otherwise only be paid if one were in a nursing home.

Common Aspects of Medicaid

- Recipients must be financially and medically in need.

- For recipients who are terminally ill, benefits go on for as long as they are ill. However, care must be provided by an agency with hospice certification and Medicaid certification.

- Payments are made directly to providers of services.

- Long-term-care costs are paid for those not covered by insurance and for patients whose finances have run out.

- Payments to foster care homes and retirement communities are not covered (except in some cases by Medicaid waiver).

- Home health care services, medical supplies, and equipment are covered.

- Eligibility is based on a person's income and assets.

- People with disabilities who are eligible for state public assistance are eligible for Medicaid.

- People with disabilities eligible for Supplemental Social Security (SSI) are eligible for Medicaid.

- In many states, there are laws (called spousal impoverishment laws) that protect a portion of the estate and assets for the healthy spouse. These come into play after other monies have been "spent down" for the care of the ill spouse. (See *General Points Regarding Asset Transfers,* p. 80.)

To find out what the benefits are, contact the local Social Security office, city or county public assistance office, or the Area Agency on Aging.

Services NOT covered by Medicaid

As a rule, Medicare, Medicaid, and private insurance do not cover many in-home services because they are not medical services. However, some community services may be called on to fill the gap for free or on a subsidized (public funding) basis. The following services usually are not covered but might be available locally free of charge:

- adult day care

- alcohol and drug programs

- case management

- household chore services
- neighborhood and local meal services, such as Meals on Wheels
- consumer protection
- transportation
- emergency response systems (which provide contact by phone or electronic device to police and rescue services)
- emergency assistance for food, clothing, or shelter
- friendly visitors (volunteers who stop by to write letters or run errands)
- services and equipment for those who have disabilities
- homemaker services
- legal and financial services
- mental health services
- respite care
- senior centers
- support groups (which will send materials if you write to them)
- telephone reassurance (volunteers who make calls to or receive calls from those who are elderly or living alone)

NOTE ➤ The U.S. Congress and the Administration made major changes to Medicare and Medicaid, which will affect payment for long-term care. As these changes are put into effect, they are posted on the Web site of the Center for Medicare and Medicaid Services (CMS): www.cms.gov

Department of Veterans Affairs Benefits

Veterans generally qualify for health services in the home if a disability is service related. Even if a disability is not service related, other benefits may be available based on income qualifications. Some states have special programs only for veterans who live in that state. Some Veterans Hospitals have programs to deliver home health care services. Contact the nearest Veterans Affairs office or veterans group in your area.

Older Americans Act and Social Services Block Grant

Some agencies that provide support services get funding under this program. Services available may include the following:

- case management and assessment
- household chore services (minor household repairs, cleaning, yard work)
- companion services
- community meals
- home-delivered hot meals (Meals on Wheels) once or twice a day
- homemaker services
- transportation

Community-Based Services

Many services are provided free by local or community groups. The groups are sometimes repaid by state, local, and federal governments, but often volunteers provide meals and social and health care services.

These services can sometimes make it possible for a person to stay at home and maintain independence.

Typical Services

Community-based services include the following:

Adult Day Care Centers, which provide services ranging from health assessment to social programs that help people with dementia or those at risk for nursing home placement.

Nutrition Sites, which serve meals in settings such as senior centers, housing projects, faith-based centers, and schools and sometimes provide transportation.

Meals on Wheels, which brings healthful food to the home.

Senior Centers, which offer a place to socialize and eat. (Often a hot meal at noontime on weekdays is the only one served.)

Transportation is offered by hospitals, nursing homes, local governments, and religious, civic, or other groups. Out-of-pocket costs vary and fees are set on a sliding scale based on ability to pay.

Do These Services Meet Your Needs?

For whatever need you have, there is most likely a program in your area. Here are some things to think about:

- Is the person the right age and income level to be eligible for the program?

- Is it necessary for the person to belong to a certain organization to be eligible?

- Is there a limit to how many times the person can use the services of the organization?

Where to Check

- local agencies (Catholic Charities, United Way, Jewish Family and Child Services, Lutheran Family Services)

- local churches, parishes, or congregations
- the government blue book pages under public service listings
- city or county public assistance offices
- rural areas (call the health agency in the county seat)
- personal doctor
- family services department
- hospital discharge planner or social worker
- insurance company
- local Area Agency on Aging
- local chapter of the National MS Society
- previous or current employer (may have benefits)
- public health department
- Social Security office
- state insurance commission
- state or local ombudsman

The Area Agency on Aging can help find services in the community. It will know whether chore services, home-delivered meals, friendly visitors, and telephone reassurance are free of charge or are provided on a sliding scale.

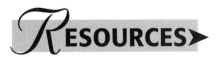

RESOURCES

AARP
601 E. Street, NW
Washington, D.C. 20049
(800) 424-3410
www.aarp.org
Provides information on Medicare beneficiaries.

Centers for Medicare and Medicaid Services

7500 Security Boulevard
Baltimore, MD 21244-1850
(800) MEDICARE (633-4227) Medicare Hotline
www.cms.gov
www.medicare.gov
Federal agency that administers the Medicare and Medicare programs, including hospice benefits.

National Association of Professional Geriatric Care Managers

1604 N. Country Club Road
Tucson, AZ 85716
(520) 881-8008
www.caremanager.org
Their Web site provides a free list of care managers in your state.

The National Council on the Aging

300 D Street SW, Suite 801
Washington, D.C. 20024
(202) 479-1200
www.ncoa.org
Provides a link to benefits (www.benefitscheckup.org) that helps seniors find state and federal benefits programs.

National Multiple Sclerosis Society

(800) FIGHT-MS (800-344-4867)
www.nationalmssociety.org
Local chapters can provide information on issues related to paying for care.

Insurance

United Seniors Council

300 D Street SW, Suite 801
Washington, D.C. 20024
(202) 479-1200
(800) 424-9046 for orders only
www.unitedseniorshealth.org

For **insurance laws and regulations,** call the state insurance department for counseling and information on the insurance laws and regulations governing your state.

Publication

Adapting: Financial Planning for a Life with Multiple Sclerosis; contact the National MS Society at (800) 344-4867 to request a copy.

If you don't have access to the Internet, ask your local library to help you locate a Web site.

Financial Management and Tax Planning

Financial Management and Tax Planning

*T*here are many legal tools and tax tips that can help you and the person in your care now and in the future. Financial and life planning is necessary and should be started early. Long-term planning will help the caregiver feel more secure, no matter what the future brings. Life planning includes looking at income tax issues, protecting existing assets, saving for the future, and planning for end of life.

You should also seek advice about insurance, employment rights, and state assistance programs. If possible, discuss all options with the person in your care.

Caregivers need to understand the coverage and policies of the person in their care. This includes any medical insurance, Medicare, Social Security benefits, and available private disability insurance. It also means knowing about their health insurance, coinsurance, copayments, deductibles, and covered expenses.

Caregivers also need to understand the Americans with Disabilities Act (ADA) and other laws that protect housing, transportation, recreation, and employment.

You should get help from legal and tax experts. Laws about estate planning can be confusing. This book does not cover them in detail but tells you about the tools available to you.

> **NOTE** Financial or estate planning is simply making sure that your property—no matter how little you have—goes to the person you choose as quickly and as cheaply as possible.

Financial Management Tools

Will—a legal document that spells out how money and property is to be given out after death. If a person is disabled or does not have the physical or mental abilities to tend to his or her own affairs, other legal papers are needed.

Living Trust—a legal document that names someone (a trustee) to manage a person's finances or assets. A trust includes advice on how to manage assets and when to distribute them (give them out). It can also protect assets from probate, which is a long legal process to make sure that the will is legal. Usually, the trust goes into effect if a person becomes unable to function well and is likely to make bad financial decisions.

Power of Attorney—a document that names someone to make decisions about money and property for a person who is unable to make those decision. A person should have one power of attorney for financial management and a separate power of attorney for health care. (See *Planning for the Life Continuum* p. 85.)

Representative Payee—someone named by the Social Security Administration to manage a person's Social Security benefits when that person is unable to look after his or her own money and bill paying.

Conservatorship—a legal proceeding in which the court names an individual to handle another's finances when that person becomes unable to do so.

Making a will, setting up a trust, providing income, and protecting assets may involve future decisions about giving to charity, insurance policies, annuities (yearly payments), and other instruments. This kind of planning is necessary and should not be put off.

NOTE Be sure to plan ahead by helping the person in your care prepare a letter of instructions. The letter should list all property and debts, location of the original will and other important documents, and names and addresses of professional advisors. It should also include funeral wishes and special instructions for giving away personal property such as furniture and jewelry.

Income Tax Considerations

In some cases, caregivers can get income tax benefits that offset their expenses as a caregiver. These tax "breaks" include claiming the person in care as a dependent and receiving a "dependent care credit." For a person who is elderly or disabled, certain tax credits also apply and some expenses are deductible.

When a Person Qualifies As a Dependent for Income Tax Purposes

A husband and wife must legally pay for each other's necessary health care, but their adult children or other relatives do not have to. However, sometimes adult children and relatives provide money or resources that will allow them to claim the person in their care as a dependent for income tax purposes.

According to the IRS, there are five tests for a person to qualify as a dependent for tax purposes:

1. The person does not earn more than a specified amount of gross income, adjusted each year to match the personal exemption. In 2005 the amount was $3,200; in 2006 it was $3,300. The exemption does not apply to a child under 19, or 24 if attending school.

2. The taxpayer provides more than one-half of the person's support.

3. The person has one of the following relationships with the taxpayer:

   - child

   - brother or sister

   - parent or grandparent

   - aunt, uncle, niece, or nephew

   - son-in-law, daughter-in-law, father-in-law, mother-in-law, brother-in-law, sister-in-law

   - a descendant of a child (grandchild, great-grandchild)

   - stepchild, stepbrother, stepsister, or stepparent

   OR

   - any person who lives in the taxpayer's home during the entire tax year and is a member of the taxpayer's household.

4. The person did not file a joint return with a spouse.

5. The person is a citizen, national, or resident of the United States, or a resident of Canada or Mexico at some time during the calendar year, or an alien child adopted by and living with a U.S. citizen.

Tax Credit for Those Who Are Elderly or Disabled

A tax credit may be available to persons who are 65 or over. It may be available to those who are permanently or totally disabled. Special rules apply for figuring out the amount of the credit. See IRS Schedule R (Form 1040) or Schedule 3 (Form 1040A).

Some life insurance policies provide tax-free benefits (accelerated death benefits), where the benefits are paid before death. Check with the life insurance company for details.

What Can Be Deducted for Income Tax Purposes

If a person can be claimed as a dependent and the caregiver itemizes, the caregiver may include medical expenses for the dependent on the caregiver's schedule of itemized deductions. If all medical expenses of the caregiver exceed 7.5% of the adjusted gross income, a deduction will be allowed.

Other deductible medical expenses are:

- improvements and additions to the home that are made for medical care purposes. (These are deductible only to the extent that they exceed the value added to the house. The entire cost of an improvement that does not increase the value of the property is deductible.)

- expenses of a dog for the blind or deaf.

- while away from home for lodging (and essential to) medical care. (The deductible expenses cannot exceed $50 per person per night. Meals are not deductible.)

- medical insurance (including premiums paid under the Social Security Act relating to supplementary medical insurance for the aged).

- long-term-care insurance premiums (subject to limitations).

- nursing homes. (The entire cost of maintenance, including meals and lodging, is deductible if the person is in a nursing home because he or she has a physical condition that requires the medical care provided.)

- transportation costs for medical care, whether around the corner or across the country. (To determine the amounts, use the actual expenses for airfare, gas, etc. If you use your own vehicle, you may use the standard deduction of eighteen cents per mile.)

See your tax preparer for rules about your exact situation.

Tip

STORING DOCUMENTS

Store—Death certificates, military records, tax returns for the last six years, pension documents

Keep in the safe-deposit box—Original will, deeds, passport, stock and bond certificates, birth and marriage certificates, insurance policies

Keep at home—a copy of the will that is in the safe deposit box

Throw out—expired insurance policies, checks that are more than one year old and are not tax-related

Funeral Expenses

Funeral expenses are not usually deducted for income tax purposes but are deducted if an estate tax return is filed.

Year-End Tax Tips for Family Caregivers

As early as possible, consider the following money-saving strategies and, if appropriate, discuss them with the person in your care.

- Pay or charge medical expenses in the year when the deduction will result in a benefit. Consider "bunching" medical deductions in one year (for example, buy January's prescription drugs in December).

- See if you qualify as head of household on the tax form.

- Consider transferring, to a beneficiary, title to the property that belongs to the person in your care. This makes sense when the beneficiary could claim ex-

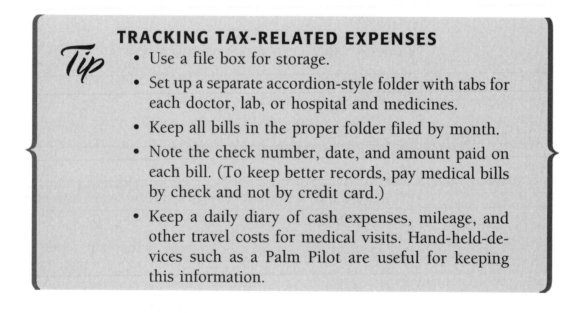

penses, such as real estate taxes, that the person in care could not claim because of a low income level.

- Determine who should pay medical bills by figuring out who will receive a tax deduction from the payment.

- Before selling assets to care for a parent, consider the tax that will have to be paid on the sale. Decide which assets have a high basis or a low basis (original purchase price), because capital gains should be kept low. Consider gifting first to the parent and having the parent sell at a lower tax rate.

- Consider giving property of the person in your care to a charity—and doing so in a way that provides a higher income each year than he or she would receive from interest on an investment.

Tip

TRACKING TAX-RELATED EXPENSES
- Use a file box for storage.
- Set up a separate accordion-style folder with tabs for each doctor, lab, or hospital and medicines.
- Keep all bills in the proper folder filed by month.
- Note the check number, date, and amount paid on each bill. (To keep better records, pay medical bills by check and not by credit card.)
- Keep a daily diary of cash expenses, mileage, and other travel costs for medical visits. Hand-held-devices such as a Palm Pilot are useful for keeping this information.

Social Security Benefits

The Social Security Administration runs two federal disability retirement programs: Social Security Disability Insurance (SSDI) and Supplemental Security Income

(SSI). SSDI is an insurance program that is funded by taxes from employees and employers. SSI is an assistance program for people with low incomes. The medical requirements and disability standards are the same.

Social Security considers a person disabled when he or she is unable to perform a paid job for which is or she is suited and the disability is expected to last for 12 months.

As a result of 2002 federal tax laws, people over 65 have no limits on the amount they can earn and still receive Social Security benefits. Call the Social Security Administration (1-800-772-1213) to get a report of your benefits record.

Understanding Social Security

- Retirement checks are loosely tied to how much a person paid into the system.

- Social Security provides the money for people who become disabled. If the person receiving Social Security dies, it also takes care of that person's spouse and children. The death benefit is $255. (📖 See *Funeral Arrangements,* p. 91.)

- Social Security typically pays $858 a month for a person who retires at 65.

- Social Security, personal savings, and employer pensions together provide financial support in old age.

> **NOTE** Name the personal representative as co-renter of the safe deposit box if the person in your care does not have a spouse or close relative. This will make it easier to get into the safe deposit box after death.

Medicaid Guidelines

The cost of nursing home care is high and can easily wipe out a couple's savings even if only one person is in a nursing home.

Currently, Medicaid rules allow a person:

- to keep a home if he or she plans to return there or if it is lived in by a spouse or a disabled or minor child

- to have a maximum individual income (which varies state to state), including pension payments and Social Security

- to have a prepaid funeral fund of $1,500

- to have a bank account of no more than $2,000

General Points Regarding Asset Transfers

- Transfers must happen at least 36 months before applying to a nursing facility. (Transfers within 36 months will delay eligibility for Medicaid. Certain transfers from trusts can delay eligibility for up to 60 months.)

- A home can be transferred within 36 months if it is transferred to a spouse, a minor, or a disabled child.

- Transfers of assets to a child may be risky if the child will not be able or willing to help the parent if extra money is needed.

- A trust may be a better option because the money is still available for the parents' needs.

- If a person sets up a special-needs trust for himself, the assets must still be spent down to qualify for Medicaid payment for nursing home care.

- Among the penalties for people who transfer assets for less than fair market value to qualify for Medicaid is a $10,000 fine and up to a year in prison.

- The healthy spouse of a person who applies for Medicaid may retain some income and resources. Each case is assessed after the applicant becomes eligible for Medicaid.

- The most individual income a person can have and still get Medicaid varies from state to state. The rules can be tricky, so seek the advice of an attorney.

Employment Planning

Employment planning and retirement tips are very important. There are many issues to look into once the person with MS can no longer work. You will need to look at sick leave, short-term disability insurance, and the Family Medical Leave Act. When the person in your care decides to stop working, you will need to look into options for medical coverage. Applying for long-term disability benefits, private and social security, can take a lot of time. You will need to find out what you can do while waiting for these new benefits.

You will also need to think about tapping into other sources of income once you decide to leave work: applying for Social Security, veterans benefits, the cash value of life insurance, long-term-care insurance; personal property, real estate, and mortgage insurance.

Abuse by Financial Advisors

Aggressive marketing to the elderly is becoming increasingly common. Although seminars for estate planning can provide useful information, they are often selling something and therefore do not offer an unbiased assessment of what a person may need. Help the person in your care avoid financial planners who may also be stock brokers or insurance agents. Before selecting a financial planner, one should always:

- Interview the financial planner and check his or her credentials (law, accounting degrees, continuing education in financial planning for the retired).

- Find out what the financial advisor will gain from your business in fee and commission income.

- Take this information into account before deciding to buy.

- Ask for the fees in writing.

- Ask if local law requires that any comparisons of plans be provided.

- Ask if the advisor is registered with the Securities and Exchange Commission.

Neither the authors nor the publisher are engaged in providing legal or tax services. This Guide is for general information only. In order to learn more about these matters, consult a CPA, attorney, or other professional advisor.

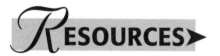 **RESOURCES**

AARP Tax-Aide
www.aarp.org/taxaide/home.htm (for a listing of site locations)
(888) 227-7669
Call 24 hours a day, 7 days a week to find a site near you. Provides free help on federal, state and local tax returns to middle- and low-income persons aged 60 years and older; also provides online counselors at the Web site. This program also accepts volunteers.

American Institute of Certified Public Accountants, Personal Financial Planning Division
www.cpapfs.org

Certified Financial Planners Board of Standards
(800) 487-1497; (303) 830-7500; (888) 237-6275
www.cfp-board.org
This organization will provide information on whether a planner is certified, how long he or she has been certified, and if any disciplinary action has ever been taken.

Financial Planning Association
Suite 400, 4100 E. Mississippi Ave.
Denver, CO 80246-3053
(800) 322-4237
Fax (404) 845-3660
www.fpanet.org
Web site provides a list and backgrounds of certified financial planners in your region and a helpful free pamphlet, Selecting a Qualified Financial Planning Professional, which lists questions you should ask a financial planner before hiring him or her.

IRS Web Site
(800) 829-3676 for publications; (800) 829-1040 for answers to tax questions
www.irs.gov
The Web site provides tax forms. Form 559 is for survivors, and Form 524 is for those who are elderly or disabled.

National Association of Personal Financial Advisors
www.napfa.org

National Multiple Sclerosis Society
(800) FIGHT-MS (800-344-4867)
www.nationalmssociety.org

Older Women's League
3300 N. Fairfax Drive, Suite 218
Arlington, VA 22201
(800) 825-3695; (703) 812-7990
Fax (703) 812-0687
www.owl-national.org

Paralyzed Veterans of America
www.pva.org
Keys to Managed Care: A Guide for People with Physical Disabilities is available at the Web site.

Social Security Administration
(800) 772-1213
www.socialsecurity.gov
Provides a personal report on a person's Social Security record. (📖 See **Funeral Arrangements,** p. 91 for details.)

Society of Financial Service Professionals
www.financialpro.org

Publication

Adapting: Financial Planning for a Life with Multiple Sclerosis. Contact the National MS Society at (800) 344-4867 to request a copy.

If you don't have home access to the Internet, ask your local library to help you locate any Web site.

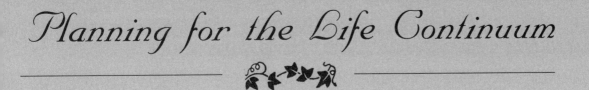

Planning for the Life Continuum

Planning for the Life Continuum

*B*esides deciding how to pay for long-term care and estate planning (topics covered in the last two chapters), it is important to decide how future health care decisions will be made **before** things reach the crisis stage. These decisions should be recorded in legal documents for two reasons:

- *to make sure that a person's wishes are honored*

- *to make sure the family has enough information about those wishes in order to make life-and-death decisions*

The ability to plan for health care decisions depends on one's ability to:

- *understand the available treatment choices*

- *understand the results of those options*

- *make and communicate a thoughtful choice*

- *express values and goals*

Once these matters are understood, a range of legal documents can be drawn up to help ensure that the person's wishes will be carried out.

The following information is not intended as legal advice. We have presented a general summary of the rights of capable adults to make, or arrange for others to make, their health care decisions. Our summary does not contain all the technical details of laws in each state. Check what your state requires by law.

Directives for Health Care

There are two types of legal documents for indicating a person's wishes for advance directives if he or she is not able to make his or her own decisions. One type outlines the kind of medical attention the person wants, and the other names the person who will make sure these wishes are carried out. (The names of the documents may be different in your state.)

Living Will

A living will spells out a person's wishes about medical care in case he or she is physically unable to state those wishes. When drawing up a living will, it is important to consider a person's attitudes and desires regarding health care. (📖 See *Special Challenges*, p. 219, for having one's wishes honored while traveling.)

Health Care Proxy (Health Care Power of Attorney or Advance Directive)

This document allows a person to name someone as a personal representative (the health care proxy or representative) and gives that person the authority, or right, to carry out the person's wishes, as outlined in the living will.

Do Not Resuscitate Order (DNR)

This document instructs medical personnel not to use CPR (cardiopulmonary resuscitation) if the person's heart stops beating.

Values History

This document explains a person's views on life and death and what he or she thinks is important. This can help the proxy or representative understand the person's wishes. It is a very helpful document because there is no way of knowing every medical situation that can possibly happen.

Why It Makes Sense to Prepare Directives

- They can be flexible and tailored to an individual's wishes.

- They apply to all health care situations.

- They may be given to anyone—a friend, relative, or spiritual advisor—to hold until needed.

- They are honored in the state where they were written and in most other states (check the state in question).

- They are not limited to issues of prolonging life but can also, for example, cover dental work and surgery.

- They can be created by filling out a standard form.

- Advance Health Care Directive forms are different from state to state and are available from most hospitals and nursing homes.

- They can be revoked (cancelled) at any time as long as the person is mentally able.

> *Tip* It is important to have these legal and health documents for the person you are caring for. It is also important that you, the caregiver, have these documents drawn up for yourself.

Hospice Care

Preparing for Hospice Care

There may come a time when you and the peson in your care explore the option of hospice care. A hospice team

Checklist **Dos and Don'ts in Planning Health Care**

✓ Do execute a new power of attorney or directive every few years to show that your wishes have not changed.

✓ Do use the proper form for your state.

✓ Do have the document drawn up by a lawyer so it follows the state rules.

✓ Do give a copy to the doctor, hospital, and any person holding power of attorney.

✓ Do ask the doctor and lawyer of the person in your care to review the document while that person is competent (mentally and physically able). Make sure they accept what is in it.

✓ Do keep a card with health care information in your wallet or that of the person in your care.

✓ Don't name the doctor as power of attorney.

✓ Do carry a copy of the document with you when you travel. (📖 See **Travel**, p. 231.)

can help ensure that the person in your care is as comfortable as possible during this period. They can also guide the person and the family's choices for final arrangements.

When an Illness Takes a Turn for the Worse

When an illness is prolonged and complex, a person will go through many physical, emotional, and spiritual changes. Some of these changes may not be too extreme, and others may be significant. Decisions to change treatment or seek alternative care may need to be made. It is best to talk about these decisions with the physicians and family of the person in your care before there is a health care crisis.

Discussing the Person's Wishes

- When possible, discuss the person's and family's wishes before an illness interferes with the person's ability to make independent decisions. Does the person have a health care proxy?

- Is there a living will or medical power of attorney?

- What would the person's choices be regarding life support?

- Would the person want to stay at home or enter a facility if it was available?

What Hospice Care Provides

Hospice has always recognized the importance including the ill person, family, and other loved ones in the care plan.

Hospice services can provide expert, kindly care and make it possible for a dying person to remain at home. The earlier hospice care begins, the more it can help and provide nonstop care. It can also help family members and friends enjoy the best quality of life possible at such a time.

Hospice is a concept of medical care that delivers comfort and support to people in the final stages of an illness—and to their families. Care is delivered by a team of specially trained medical professionals who focus on easing pain and managing symptoms. They provide medical, emotional, psychological, and spiritual care to the person and family and assist the family in coping with their coming loss and their grief afterwards.

Most hospice care is delivered in the home but can also be provided in hospice and other care facilities. The person who is ill and the family are the core of the hospice team and are at the center of all decision making.

Here are some questions you can ask in selecting hospice care:

- Is the agency licensed, and accredited by a nationally recognized organization?

- Are they Medicare certified?

- What are their billing policies and payment plans?

- Can they provide references, such as local hospital and care centers, institutions, and care givers?

- How do they evaluate the individual's readiness for hospice care?

- How are their caregivers supervised?

- What are their expectations of the family in sharing in caregiving?

- Are you comfortable with the program? Does it feel like the right fit?

Funeral Arrangements

Although an uncomfortable topic, it is helpful for the family to discuss all aspects of death and all funeral arrangements while the person is still alive. This will ensure that the wishes of the individual are carried out with a minimum of cost and decrease the stress on the family at the time of death. The simpler the service, the less expensive it will be, but remember that ritual is important to a bereaved family. Contact funeral homes in your area for specific details.

If your area has a nonprofit memorial association, its volunteers have likely done price comparisons of local funeral homes.

NOTE People often place their funeral instructions in a safe-deposit box that is not to be opened until after the funeral. Keep the instructions where they can be easily located and give a copy to the nearest relative.

Information That Will Be Needed After Death

Many facts can be gathered in a person's lifetime and recorded in a simple estate planner booklet. Keep this booklet or form (available from most funeral homes, some attorneys, and stationery stores) in a safe place and let the family know where it is located.

Be sure you have telephone numbers for the following people so you can reach them easily:

- accountant
- attorney
- business associates
- clergy
- doctor
- employees
- employer
- estate executor or trustee
- family
- financial advisor
- friends
- funeral home where the funeral is preplanned
- health representative, if other than you
- tax preparer

Financial Information to Record in the Estate Planner

In an estate planning booklet or informal list, keep clear records of the following information, complete with account numbers, addresses, telephone numbers, and the location of the documents:

- investments, their amounts, and brokers
- annuities
- bank checking and savings accounts
- life insurance with policy numbers
- Medicare and supplemental insurance
- military service and veterans' benefits
- mortgages and liabilities
- pension plans, profit-sharing, Keogh plans, and IRAs
- real estate holdings
- safe-deposit box location and key
- Social Security card and number and the date benefits began, if applicable
- workers compensation, if applicable
- list of motor vehicles owned and location of titles

Survivors' Benefits

Carefully check all life and casualty insurance and death benefits. Check on income for survivors from a credit union, trade union, fraternal organization, the military, and the Social Security Administration. Some debts and installment payments may carry insurance clauses that will cancel them. Consult with creditors if there will be a delay in payments and ask for more time.

Social Security Benefits

The widow, dependent widower, children, and dependent parents of an insured person may be eligible for monthly survivors' payments. (They usually don't start for about six weeks). However, Social Security benefits are not paid automatically. To apply, you will need the following documents:

- birth certificate of the deceased

- marriage certificate

- birth certificates of survivors (under 22 years of age if they are full-time college students; under 18 if they are not)

- proof of widow's or widower's age, if 62 or older

- proof of termination of any preceding marriage

- record of income for the preceding year

The surviving spouse or minor children may also receive a modest one-time death benefit. Ask your Social Security office for help in filling out your claims.

A personalized **Social Security report**, which outlines benefits, earnings history, and other useful information can be obtained by calling (800) 772-1213.

If you have an e-mail address, you can obtain an electronic estimate of Social Security retirement and disability benefits, as well as benefits paid to the survivors, by signing on to the Web site http://www.ssa.gov. It will not include a complete earnings history. You must know the person's name, Social Security number, date of birth, place of birth, and mother's maiden name.

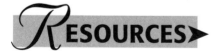

RESOURCES

Administration on Aging
www.aoa.gov/legal/hotline.html
Web site lists legal hotlines for the states that have them for those 60 and older.

The Equal Justice Network

www.equaljustice.org/hotline
A Web site sponsored by programs in the field offering legal advice over the telephone.

Funeral Consumers Alliance

33 Patchen Road
South Burlington, VT 05403
(800) 765-0107
www.funerals.org
Provides information about alternatives for funeral or non-funeral dispositions; can refer you to individual societies in the state of your choice.

Funeral Service Consumer Assistance Program

P.O. Box 486
Elm Grove, WI 53122-0486
(800) 662-7666
www.fsef.org
Provides help to consumers and funeral directors to resolve disagreements about funeral service contracts; provides referrals and information on death, grief, and funeral service.

Hospice Foundation of America

1621 Connecticut Avenue NW, #300
Washington, DC 20009
(800) 854-3402
www.hospicefoundation.org
Provides information and referral service, resources on end-of-life care, search engine to end-of-life Web sites, free brochures on hospice, volunteering, and bereavement.

Last Acts

www.lastacts.org
Comprehensive Web site with links to resources for end-of-life care.

National Hospice and Palliative Care Organization
(703) 243-5900
Hotline (800) 658-8898
www.nhpco.org
Provides information on hospice, referrals to local hospices, and outreach hospice services to families of dying people.

National Multiple Sclerosis Society
(800) FIGHT-MS (800-344-4867)
www.nationalmssociety.org

Public Reference Branch
Federal Trade Commission
Sixth Street & Pennsylvania Avenue, N.W.
Washington, D. C. 20580
For the free brochure Facts for Consumers: Funerals—a Consumer Guide, *send a self-addressed, stamped envelope.*

Call your local **Social Security Administration, State Health Department, State Hospice Organization**, or call 1-800-633-4227 **Medicare Hotline** to learn about hospice benefits.

Publication

Adapting: Financial Planning for a Life with Multiple Sclerosis. Contact the National Multiple Sclerosis Society at (800) FIGHT-MS (800-344-4867) to request a copy.

If you don't have access to the Internet, ask your local library to help you locate any Web site.

Preparing the Home

Preparing the Home

It may be necessary to make some changes to your home. Most families find that they do not have to redesign their home. It is important, however, to look at one's home with an eye towards saving energy, making work easier to do, and making the home more accessible (easier for the person in your care to use). It is better to make changes sooner rather than later.

We believe it is important for our readers to be aware of the "ideal" as they plan the changes they will make. If you are thinking of buying a new home, use these guidelines to help choose the right home that will meet future needs.

Adapting for Safety, Accessibility, and Comfort

The main goal in any home is safety. You and the person in your care need to take a close look at your home. You may also want to ask the advice of a friend or relative.

> **NOTE** Leave a blanket, pillow, and phone on the floor; however, not in the flow of foot traffic. In case of a fall, the person in your care can stay warm and call for help.

As you plan for safety in the home, consider what you need now and what you will need in the future. For example, furniture that works well now may need to be changed or replaced later when the person can no longer get up from low seats. Your main goal is to make the home as safe as possible.

As you make changes to the home, don't forget your own comfort and ease. Making life easier for yourself means you will have more time to provide care or to rest. In the long run, this will improve the overall setting for care.

The Home Environment

The ideal home for a person with MS is on one level (ground floor). Having more than one floor is all right only if there is an elevator or another approved lift device, or if the person with MS does not need to go to the second floor. The ideal care home is laid out in such a way that the caregiver and the person in care can see each other from other rooms.

Safety

For the safest home, follow as many of these steps as possible:

- Remove all furniture that is not needed.

- Place the remaining furniture so that there is enough space for a walker or wheelchair. This will avoid the need for a person who is elderly or disabled to move around coffee tables and other barriers. Move any low tables that are in the way.

- Once the person in your care has gotten used to where the furniture is, do not change it.

- Make sure furniture will not move if leaned on.

- Ensure that the armrests of a favorite chair are long enough to help the person get up and down.

- Modify or cushion sharp corners on furniture, cabinets, and vanities.

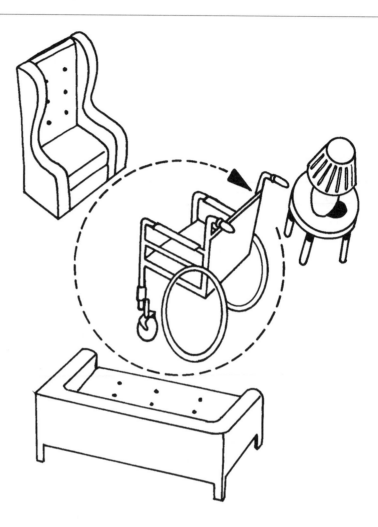

► *To accommodate a wheelchair, arrange furniture 5¹/₂ feet apart.*

- Make chair seats 20″ high. (Wood blocks or a wooden platform can be placed under large, heavy furniture to raise it to this level.)

- Have a carpenter put railings in places where a person might need extra support. (Using a carpenter can ensure that railings will bear a person's full weight and will not give way.)

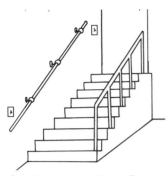

▲ *Always provide railings along stairways. When possible, extend the handrail past the bottom and top step.*

▶ *Place nonskid tape on the edges of steps.*

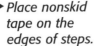
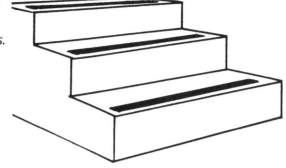

- Place masking or colored tape on glass doors and picture windows.

- Use automatic night-lights in the rooms used by the person in your care.

- Clear fire-escape routes.

- Put smoke alarms on every floor and outside every bedroom.

- Place a fire extinguisher in the kitchen.

- Consider the need for monitors and intercoms.

- Place nonskid tape on the edges of stairs. (Consider painting the edge of the first and last step a different color from the floor.)

- Thin-piled carpet is easier to walk on than thick pile. Avoid "busy" patterns.

NOTE ▶ For a safer home setting for a person with a respiratory (breathing) condition such as asthma, emphysema, or chronic bronchitis, avoid the following:

- rugs
- belt-type humidifiers
- overstuffed furniture
- books and book shelves
- pets and stuffed toys

- pleated lampshades
- dirty heat ducts and air filters
- tobacco smoke
- wool blankets and clothing

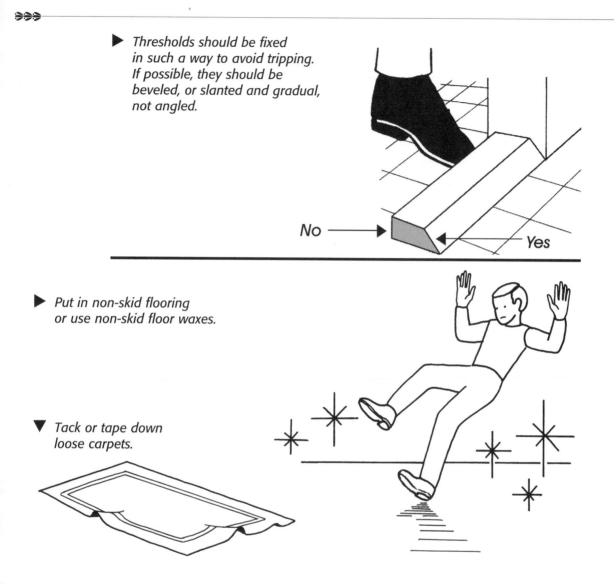

▶ Thresholds should be fixed in such a way to avoid tripping. If possible, they should be beveled, or slanted and gradual, not angled.

No ⟶   ⟵ Yes

▶ Put in non-skid flooring or use non-skid floor waxes.

▼ Tack or tape down loose carpets.

- Be sure stairs have an even surface with no metal strips or rubber mats that can cause tripping.

- Remove anything that might lead to tripping.

- Secure electrical and telephone cords to walls.

- Adjust or remove rapidly closing doors.

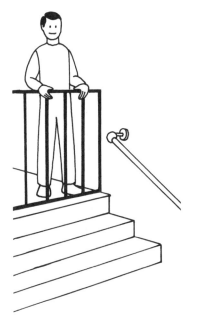

▲ *A safety gate at the top of stairs can prevent falls.*

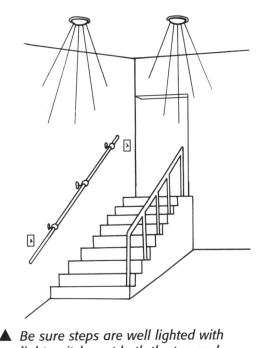

▲ *Be sure steps are well lighted with light switches at both the top and bottom of the stairs.*

- Place protective screens on fireplaces.

- Cover exposed hot water pipes.

- Provide plenty of indirect no-glare lighting.

- Place light switches next to room entrances so the lights can be turned on before entering a room. Consider "clap-on" lamps beside the bed.

- Use 100–200 watt lightbulbs for close-up activities (but make sure lamps can handle the extra wattage).

NOTE Contrasting colors play a big part in seeing well. As much as possible, the color of furniture, toilet seats, counters, etc., should be different from the floor color.

- Plan for extra outdoor lighting for good nighttime visibility, especially on stairs and walkways.

- If possible, install a carbon monoxide (CO) detector that sounds an alarm when dangerous levels of CO are reached. Call the **American Lung Association** at 1-800-LUNG USA for details.

- Develop an emergency evacuation plan in case of fire.

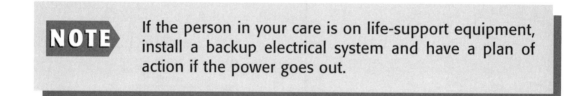

NOTE If the person in your care is on life-support equipment, install a backup electrical system and have a plan of action if the power goes out.

Comfort and Convenience

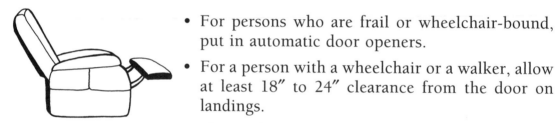

- For persons who are frail or wheelchair-bound, put in automatic door openers.

- For a person with a wheelchair or a walker, allow at least 18″ to 24″ clearance from the door on landings.

- Plan to leave enough space (a minimum of 32″ clear) for moving a hospital bed and wheelchair through doorways.

▲ *Think about getting a power-assisted recliner that allows the power-assist feature to be turned off.*

▶ *Install entry ramps. Rails can be added for more safety. Ramps should not rise more than 1″ per foot, and should be 30–40″ wide.*

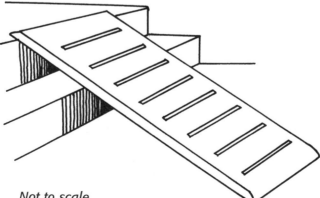

Not to scale

> **NOTE** ▷ If you are redoing a two-story house or building a new one, have the contractor frame in the shell of the elevator and then add the elevator unit later if needed. Use the space as a closet now.

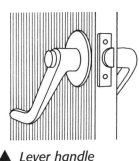

▲ *Lever handle*

- To widen doorways, remove the molding and replace regular door hinges with offset hinges. Whenever possible, remove doors.

- Install lever handles on all doors.

- If a person who is disabled must be moved from one story to another, install a stair elevator.

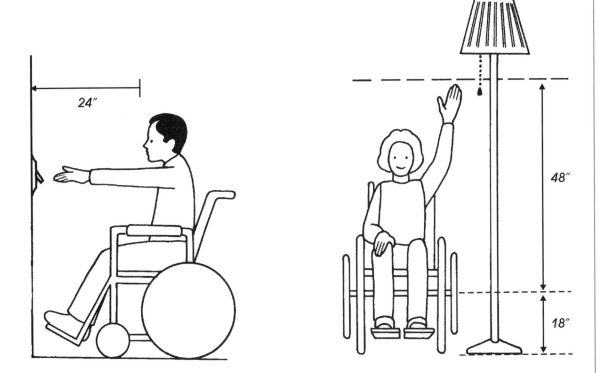

▲ *A person can reach forward about 24" from a seated position. Between 18" and 48" from the floor is the ideal position for light switches, telephones, and mailboxes.*

The Bathroom

Many accidents happen in bathrooms, so check the safety of the bathroom that you will use for home care.

Safety

▶ Install grab bars beside and in back of the toilet, along the edge of the sink, and in the tub and shower according to the needs of each person.

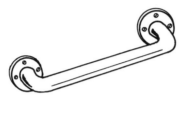

▶ Five-inch door pulls or utility handles can be put on door frames and window sills.

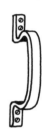

Safety

- Cover all sharp edges with rubber cushioning.
- Install lights in medicine cabinets so mistakes are not made when taking medicine.
- Remove locks on bathroom doors.
- Use nonskid safety strips or a nonslip bath mat in the tub or shower.
- Consider installing a grab rail on the edge of the vanity. (Do not use a towel bar.)
- Remove glass shower doors or replace them with unbreakable plastic.
- Use only electrical appliances with a ground fault interrupted (GFI) feature.
- Install GFI electrical outlets.
- Set the hot water thermostat below 120° F.
- Use faucets that mix hot and cold water, or paint hot water knobs and faucets red.

- Insulate hot water pipes to prevent burns.
- Install toilet guard rails or provide a portable toilet seat with built-in rails. (📖 See *Equipment and Supplies,* p. 117.)

Comfort and Convenience

- If possible, have the bathroom in a straight path from the bedroom of the person in your care.
- Install a ceiling heat lamp.
- Place a telephone near the toilet.
- Provide soap-on-a-rope or put a bar of soap in the toe of a nylon stocking and tie it to the grab bar.
- Place toilet paper within easy reach.
- Try to provide enough space for two people at the bathroom sink.
- If possible, have the sink 32″ to 34″ from the floor.
- Use levers instead of handles on the faucets.
- Provide a raised (elevated) toilet seat.

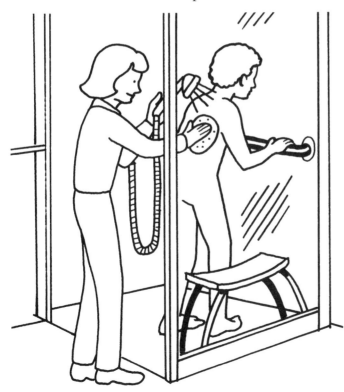

◀ *If possible, have a shower stall that is large enough for two people. Use a hand-held shower head with a very long hose and adjustable jet stream. Put a tub seat or bench in the shower stall.*

> **NOTE** Place frequently used items at a level between the shoulders and knees. This will reduce the chance of falls and avoid reaching and bending.

The Bedroom

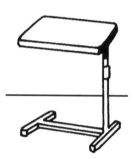

▲ *Provide an adjustable over-the-bed table like the ones used to serve meals in hospital rooms.*

Ideally provide three bedrooms—one for the person in care, one for yourself, and one for the home health aide. Also—

- Install a monitor to listen to activity in the room of the person in your care. (Some are inexpensive and portable.)

- Make the bedroom bright and cheerful.

- Make sure adequate heat (65° F at night) and fresh air are available.

- Provide a firm mattress.

- Provide TV and radio.

- Consider a fish aquarium for distraction and relaxation.

- Use disposable pads to protect furniture.

- Install room-darkening blinds or shades.

- Place closet rods 48″ from the floor.

- Provide a chair for dressing.

- Keep a flashlight at the bedside table.

- Provide a bedside commode with a 4″ foam pad on the seat for comfort.

- Hang a bulletin board with pictures of family and friends where it can be easily seen.

- Provide a sturdy chair or table next to the bed for help getting in and out of bed.

- Make the bed 22″ high and stabilize it against a wall. Or use a bed with wheels that can be locked. This will allow the person who uses it to get up and down safely.

- Use blocks to raise a bed's height, but be sure to stabilize them carefully.

▶ *Bedside commode and bed with trapeze bar*

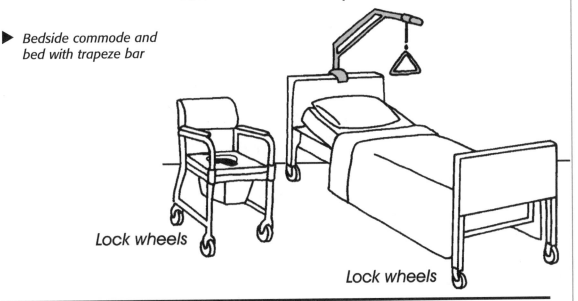

Lock wheels

Lock wheels

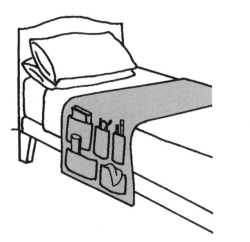

▲ *Make a bed organizer to hold facial tissues, lotion, and other items needed at the bedside. Do this by attaching pockets to a large piece of fabric spread across the bed.*

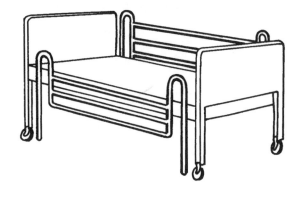

▲ *If all the care is at the bedside, consider a hospital bed. This will be helpful for both you and the person in your care.*

The Telephone

Contact your local phone company's special-needs department or visit a store that sells phones and accessories to inquire about—

- increasing the number size on your phone dial for improved visibility and ease of use

▶ *Telephone with enlarged numbers*

- a phone cradle
- step-by-step, large-size instructions for using the phone
- amplified handsets
- signal devices, such as lights that flash when a call is coming in
- TTY (text telephone yoke), a device for people with hearing loss
- a portable phone
- speed-dial buttons with names or pictures of friends and family instead of numbers
- a one-line phone that automatically connects to a preset number when the button is pressed
- a list of emergency numbers and medicines beside the telephone (📖 See *Setting Up a Plan of Care,* p. 141, for a sample)

- clear instructions on how to direct emergency personnel to the street address of the house

- a personal emergency response system to signal a friend or emergency service

NOTE Some communities provide a free telephone reassurance service. TRS will make a brief, daily telephone call to persons who are elderly or disabled to reassure them and to share crime prevention information. Call your local police department.

Outdoor Areas

Safe outdoor areas are important. Outdoor safety features should include:

- ramps for access on uneven ground

- a deck with a sturdy railing

- outside doors that are locked or have alarms

- a hidden key outside

- enough light to see walkways at night

- nonslip step surfaces in good repair

- stair handrails fastened to their fittings

- step edges marked with reflective paint

In addition, unplug or remove power tools.

Additional Considerations

It is important to find out how many levels of living space there are inside and outside your home. Note any possible access problems. Canes, crutches, and walkers need a certain amount of open space for moving around and turning. Wheelchairs and scooters require a wide turning area.

You and the person in your care need to think about your activities at home. Ask who, what, where, when, why, and how about everything you do. Who can help with what specific jobs? What jobs can you get rid of or make simpler? Would you be more comfortable doing the job somewhere else? Can you make the home more pleasant? In terms of work centers, plan where you can sit for each of your activities so that everything you need is at hand. Ask for input from everyone in the family. Making work simpler will help the person with MS and can save time as well.

If Changes Are Needed

Changing certain things can increase safety, accessibility, and comfort for everyone. But before making major changes to the home, ask a doctor for a referral to an occupational therapist (OT) for a home visit. An OT can recommend ways to keep the person with MS as independent as possible, ensure safety, and reduce the physical strain on the caregiver. Ramps, wider doorways, and repairs in the kitchen and bath can often solve accessibility problems. Not all changes are major expenses.

Almost any equipment or installation required by a disability can be tax deductible, within IRS rules and guidelines.

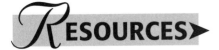

RESOURCES

Check with local police to find out if they manage a **Senior Locks Program**. This is a program whereby home-owners 55 and older who meet federal income guidelines can have deadbolt locks and other security devices installed at no charge.

AARP
601 E Street, NW
Washington, DC 20049
(800) 424-3410
www.aarp.org
Call or write for the booklet The Do-Able, Renewable Home. *Members can receive one copy at no charge.*

Center for Universal Design
North Carolina State University
Box 8613
Raleigh, NC 27695-8613
(919) 515-3082 (V/TTY) Fax (919) 515-3023
(800) 647-6777
www.design.ncsu.edu\cud
E-mail: cud@ncsu.edu
Established to improve the quality and availability of housing for people with disabilities. Services include information, referral service, training and education, technical design assistance, and publications.

Metropolitan Center for Independent Living, Inc. (MCIL)
1600 University Avenue West, Suite 16
St. Paul, MN 55104-3825
(651) 603-2029
www.wheelchairramp.org
E-mail: jimwi@mcil-mn.org
Web site features How to Build Wheelchair Ramps for Homes, *an online manual for the design and construction of wheelchair ramps.*

National Association of Home Builders Research Center
(800) 638-8556; (301) 249-4000
www.nahbrc.org
Call for its book A Comprehensive Approach to Retrofitting Houses for a Lifetime, *$15 plus postage and handling.*

National Institute for Rehabilitation Engineering
P.O. Box 1088
Hewett, NJ 07421
(800) 736-2216; (973) 853-6585 Fax (928) 832-2894
www.theoffice.net/nire
E-mail: nire@theoffice.net

National Multiple Sclerosis Society
(800) FIGHT-MS (800-344-4867)
www.nationalmssociety.org
Chapters have information on equipment discounts, entitlement programs, and local resources.

Paralyzed Veterans of America
801 18th Street NW
Washington, DC 20006-3517
Tel: 1-800-424-8200
www.pva.org
Not just for veterans, not just for paralysis. Ask for the Architecture Program.

Publication

At Home with MS: Adapting Your Environment, by Jane E. Harmon, OTR
Contact the National Multiple Sclerosis Society at (800) FIGHT-MS (800-344-4867) to request a copy or visit www.nationalmssociety.org

If you don't have access to the Internet, ask your local library to help you locate a Web site.

Equipment and Supplies

Equipment and Supplies

*T*o provide proper at-home care, you will need certain supplies. There are two types:

- *general medical supplies*
- *durable medical equipment*

Before buying anything or signing a rental contract, ask your doctor, physical or occupational therapist, or nurse. Salespeople may not be trained to assess what the person in your care may need. Occupational therapists can advise you on low-cost substitutes for expensive equipment. With the proper doctor's orders (referrals) and documentation, some equipment is covered by Medicare or private insurance. Get in touch with your insurance carrier to see if what you need is covered and follow the company's rules for getting approval before buying.

Where to Buy Needed Supplies

Buy medical equipment and supplies from dealers that are well established and that are well known for good service. Be sure to get advice about where to buy from your health care professionals or hospital discharge planner. To compare prices, use the chart on page 133.

Look in the Yellow Pages under Surgical Appliances, Physicians and Surgeons, Equipment & Supplies, and First Aid Supplies. Sources include

- surgical supply stores
- pharmacies

- hospitals
- home health care agencies
- medical supply catalogs

Where to Borrow

For short-term use, think about borrowing equipment from the following local groups:

- National Multiple Sclerosis Society
- Salvation Army
- Red Cross
- Visiting Nurses Association
- home health care agencies
- National Easter Seal Society
- charity organizations
- faith-based groups, senior centers, leisure clubs

NOTE Never buy equipment from someone who calls you on the phone to sell you a product. Do not buy from a door-to-door salesperson. Do not buy from someone who calls you even before you know what equipment will be needed.

Checklist *General Supplies**

- ✓ antibacterial hand cleaner (kills germs)
- ✓ bacteriostatic ointment (stops the growth of germs)
- ✓ bandages, gauze pads, tape
- ✓ blankets (2 or 3)
- ✓ cotton balls and swabs
- ✓ toothbrush, toothpaste
- ✓ denture or dental care items
- ✓ kidney-shaped basin for oral care
- ✓ container for disposing of syringes (needles)
- ✓ disposable Chux underpad that keeps moisture out, for bed protection
- ✓ draw sheets for use in turning someone in bed
- ✓ finger towels and washcloths
- ✓ foam rubber pillows
- ✓ head pillows
- ✓ heating pad
- ✓ hydrogen peroxide
- ✓ ice bag
- ✓ lotion

- ✓ 4 bed sheets (at least)
- ✓ oral laxative
- ✓ poster with first aid procedures
- ✓ pressure pad and pump
- ✓ sterile rubber gloves
- ✓ rubbing alcohol
- ✓ seat belts (to prevent sliding down in a chair)
- ✓ shower cap
- ✓ soap for dry skin
- ✓ thermometers (rectal and oral)
- ✓ tissues
- ✓ disposable underpants
- ✓ incontinence briefs
- ✓ panty liners
- ✓ toilet paper tongs to take care of personal hygiene
- ✓ waterproof sheeting
- ✓ roll belt restraint
- ✓ gait/transfer belt
- ✓ Medic Alert® identification

*As needed.

How to Pay

If you need assistance in paying for medical equipment:

- Ask the doctor to write an order for a home evaluation (assessment), including an evaluation of needed equipment.

- Find out if the equipment is partly or completely covered by private health insurance with home care benefits.

- Check state retirement and union programs.

Medicare does not help pay for assistive devices, but does pay for durable medical equipment in some cases. To be covered, the equipment must be prescribed by a doctor and it must be medically necessary. It must be useful only to the sick or injured person and must be reusable. Medicare will pay for the rental of certain items for no more than 15 months. After that time you may buy the equipment from the supplier. If the person in your care has met the deductible, Medicare will pay 80% of the approved charges on the rental, purchase, and service of equipment that the doctor has ordered.

GETTING ORGANIZED
Keep supplies together that are used often and keep a list of supplies so you can easily replace them.

Be prepared for emergencies. Have on hand a flashlight, a battery-run radio, a battery-run clock, fresh batteries, extra blankets, candles with holders, matches, and a manual can opener.

Medical Equipment

You will need to have special equipment for different rooms in the house, as well as equipment to increase the person's ability to get around.

Equipment for the Bedroom

The equipment you need to have depends on the person's medical condition. This equipment might include some of the items listed below.

- **hospital bed**—allows positioning (adjusting) that is not possible in a regular bed and aids in resting and breathing more comfortably and getting in and out of bed more easily

- **alternating pressure mattress**—reduces pressure on skin tissue

- **egg-carton pad**—a foam mattress pad shaped like the bottom of an egg carton that reduces pressure and improves air circulation

- **portable commode chair**—for ease of toileting at the bedside

- **trapeze bar**—provides support and a secure hand-hold while changing positions

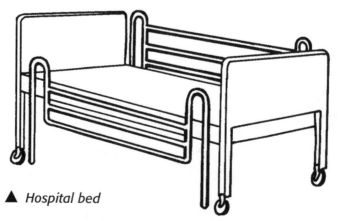

▲ *Hospital bed*

- **transfer board**—a smooth board for independent or assisted transfer from bed to wheelchair, toilet, or portable commode (📖 See p. 286)

- **hydraulic lift**—for use on a person who is difficult to move

- **over-the-bed table**—provides a surface for eating, reading, writing, and game playing (could be an adjustable ironing board)

- **mechanical or electric lift chair**—for help getting up from a chair

- **blanket support**—a wire support that keeps heavy bed linens off injured areas or the feet

- **urinal and bed pan**—for toileting in the bed

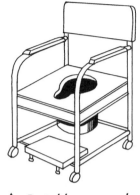

▲ *Portable commode chair*

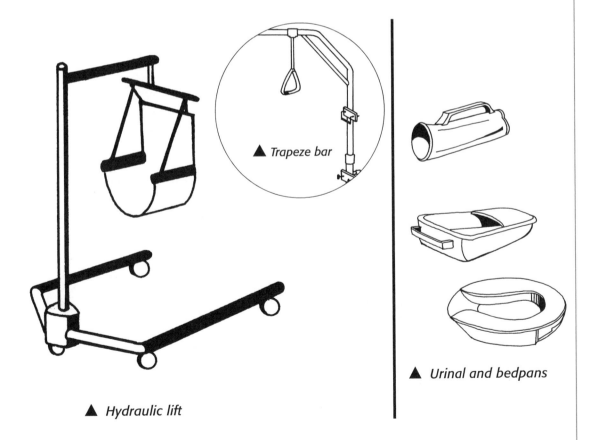

▲ *Trapeze bar*

▲ *Urinal and bedpans*

▲ *Hydraulic lift*

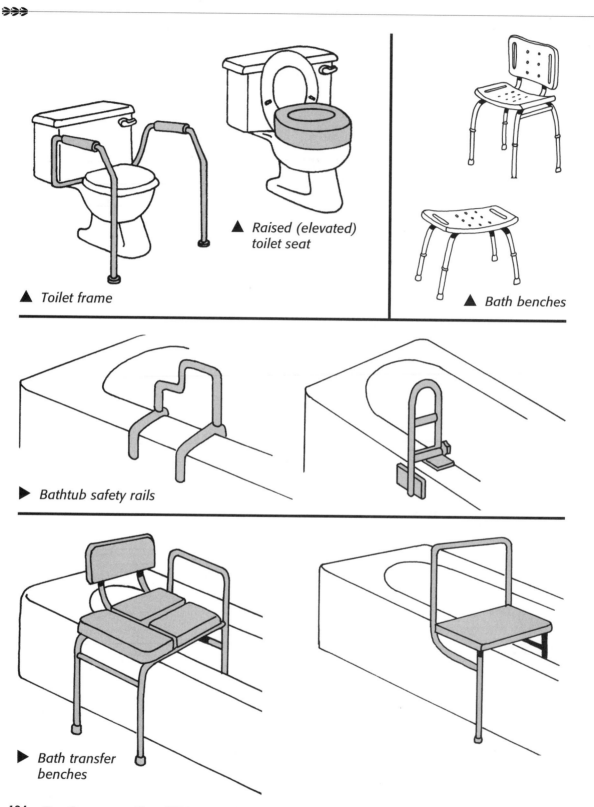

▲ Toilet frame

▲ Raised (elevated) toilet seat

▲ Bath benches

▶ Bathtub safety rails

▶ Bath transfer benches

Equipment for the Bathroom

The equipment you will need depends on the person's needs. You should consider providing the following:

- **raised (elevated) toilet seat**—used to assist a person who has difficulty getting up or down on a toilet (available in molded plastic and clamp-on models for different toilet bowl styles)

- **commode aid**—a device that acts as an elevated toilet seat when used with a splash guard, or as a commode when used with a pail

- **toilet frame**—a free-standing unit that fits over the toilet and provides supports on either side for ease in getting up and down

- **grab bars for tub and shower**—properly installed wall-mounted safety bars that hold a person's weight

- **safety mat and strips**—rough vinyl strips that stick to the bottom of the tub and shower to prevent slipping

- **hand-held shower hose**—a movable shower hose and head that allows the water to be directed to all parts of the body

- **bath bench**—aid for a person who has difficulty sitting down in or getting up from the bottom of the tub

- **bath transfer bench**—a bench that goes across the side of the tub and allows a person to get out of the tub easily

- **bathtub safety rails**—support for getting in and out of the tub

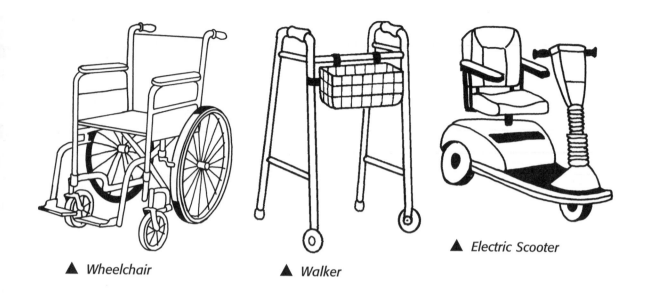

▲ Wheelchair   ▲ Walker   ▲ Electric Scooter

Mobility Aids

Mobility aids include devices that help a person move around without help. They also help the caregiver transfer the person in and out of bed and from bed to a chair.

They include—

- a wheelchair with padding and removable arms

- a walker to help maintain balance and provide some support

- a 3- or 4-wheel electric scooter

- crutches when weight cannot be put on one leg or foot

- a cane to provide light weight-bearing support

- a transfer board (9″ x 24″) for moving someone in and out of bed (📖 See illustration p. 290)

- a gait/transfer belt (📖 See how to use on p. 286)

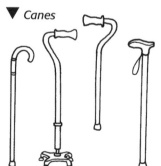

▼ Canes

Wheelchair Requirements

Proper fit, as determined by a physical therapist.

- safety
- durability
- ease of repair
- attractive appearance
- comfort
- ease of handling
- cushions

Wheelchair Attachments

- a brake lever extension on the handle
- elevated leg rests and removable footrests
- armrests that can be taken off

 NOTE Some states have lemon laws that cover wheelchairs and other assistive devices. If you think there is something wrong with the equipment you have bought and you want to find out if it qualifies as a lemon, call the Attorney General's office in your state. They may be able to help you in getting a replacement or a refund.

Assistive Devices

For those with poor sight and hearing or other limitations, there are many aids to make life easier. Look into all the options and you will find that your job as caregiver becomes easier too.

Sight Aids

- prism glasses
- magnifying glasses
- prescription glasses
- Braille books and signs
- cassette players and books on tape
- telesensory devices that change printed letters into symbols that can be touched

Listening Aids

- hearing aids (order from an audiologist, or hearing therapist, who allows a free 30-day trial and is a registered dealer)
- sound systems that amplify (make louder)
- telephone amplifiers (for increased volume)
- devices for getting close-captioned TV programs

Tip **HELP FOR SPECIAL EQUIPMENT**
Look into whether Medicaid or the Lion's Club in your state can pay for hearing aids.

Eating Aids

- spoons that swivel for those who have trouble with wrist movement

- foam that can be fit over utensils to increase the gripping surface so they can be lifted more easily

- plate guards or dishes with high sides that make it easier to scoop food onto a spoon

- rocker knives that can cut food with a rocking motion

- food-warming dishes for slow eaters

- mugs with two handles, a cover, a spout, and a suction base

▼ *Eating aids—mug, utensils with built-up handles, food guard, one-hand knife, swivel spoon*

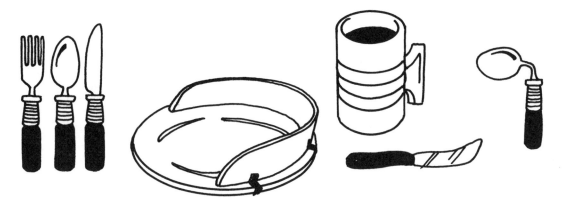

Dressing Aids

- button hooks that make buttoning clothes easy

- dressing sticks that make it possible to dress without bending

- long-handled shoehorns so a person doesn't have to bend over when putting on shoes

- sock aids that keep stockings open while they are being put on

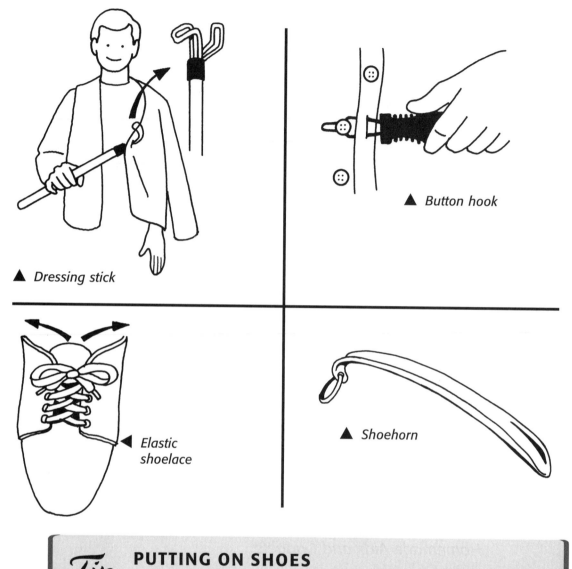

▲ Dressing stick

▲ Button hook

◀ Elastic shoelace

▲ Shoehorn

> *Tip*
>
> **PUTTING ON SHOES**
> For people who have trouble tying laces, turn a lace-up shoe into a slip-on by replacing the cotton shoelaces with elastic ones.

Devices for Summoning Help

- touch-tone phones with speed dials

- medical security response systems
- beepers for the caregiver

Cooling Devices

Heat can be the enemy for many people with MS. Learning how to "cool it!" in the summer months can be a problem. Fortunately, there are a number of cooling devices available to help the caregiver or person with MS beat the heat:

- There are scarves and neck wraps that can be made cool by simply soaking in water.
- Cooling vests are another staple among cooling devices.
- There are devices for cooling wrists and ankles. One brand has arm and leg bands made of terrycloth into which you insert custom-size freezer packs.

Computer Equipment

There are countless hardware and software programs to make computers easier for people with disabilities to use. Alternative keyboards, puff switches for those who cannot use a mouse, screen readers, talking word processors, and voice recognition software are available today.

Homemade Aids and Gadgets

- wrist straps for canes—tape tied on a cane so it can be hung from the wrist while walking upstairs
- bicycle baskets—strapped to a walker to store necessities and leave the hands free
- an egg carton—to organize pills
- rubber safety mats—ideal for the tub, shower, or any slippery surface; also useful to make place on trays and tables for a nonslip surface

- key—put the end of the key that you hold into a large cork for ease of grip

- foot-operated door levers—made by attaching rope to a "stirrup" and tying it to the lever handle

- language tags—cardboard tags with words that can be used to express needs

- light-switch enlargements—made by putting a rubber pen cap over a light switch

- enlarged pull switches—made by putting a plastic ball over small switches

- clips for canes—spring clips or Velcro® placed on favorite chairs to keep a cane from falling

- bedside rails—wooden rails attached to the floor at right angles on swivel hinges

- pull rope—rope attached to the footboard of the bed to help someone change positions in bed

Equipment Cost-Comparison Chart *(Example)*

Item	Purchase Price	Rental Fee × Months Needed	Covered by Medicare Yes/No	Vendor
bath stool	$			
bed pan				
bed safety accessories				
cane				
commode				
crutches				
hospital bed				
mattress				
oxygen				
raised toilet seat				
special equipment				
trapeze				
walker				
wheelchair				
3- or 4-wheel scooter				
other				
Totals	$			

Specialized Hospital-Type Equipment

- **oxygen tanks**, for use when oxygen is needed as a medication

- **breathing tube (transtracheal oxygen therapy equipment)**, for use when oxygen is delivered into the lungs through a flexible tube that goes from the neck directly into the trachea (sometimes called the windpipe)

- **compressors and hand-held nebulizers (inhalers)**, which reduce medication to a form that can be inhaled

- **suction catheters**, which clear mucus and secretions from the back of the throat when someone cannot swallow

- **home infusion equipment**, or IV (intravenous) therapy, which delivers antibiotics, blood products, chemotherapy, hydration (water), pain management, parenteral (IV) nutrition, and specialty medications

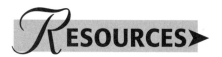

ABLEDATA
8630 Fenton Street, Suite 930
Silver Spring, MD 20910-3319
(800) 227-0216; (301) 608-8998; Fax (301) 608-8958
www.abledata.com
Stores information on thousands of assistive devices for home health care, from eating utensils to wheelchairs. Provides prices, names, and addresses of suppliers.

AbilityHub
www.abilityhub.com
Assistive technology for people who have difficulty operating a computer.

Adaptive Environments Center Inc.
374 Congress Street, Suite 301
Boston, MA 02210
(617) 695-1225 (v/tty); Fax (617) 482-8099
www.adaptiveenvironments.org
E-mail: info@adaptiveenvironments.org

Alliance for Technology Access
www.ataccess.org
A network of community-based resource centers, developers, vendors, and associates dedicated to providing information and support services to children and adults with disabilities, and increasing their use of standard, assistive, and information technologies. You can order their book Computer Resources for People with Disabilities *online.*

American Occupational Therapy Association (AOTA)
4720 Montgomery Lane
P.O. Box 31220
Bethesda, MD 20824-1220
(301) 652-2682; Fax (301) 652-7711
www.aota.org
Provides consumer publications.

Apple Computer Accessibility
www.apple.com/accessibility
Committed to helping people with disabilities to access their computers.

AT&T Special Needs Center
Tel: (800) 872-3883 (TTY)
Provides free directory assistance (with an application) and operator's help dialing for those who are vision impaired and disabled.

Briggs
(800) 247-2343

Independent Living Research Utilization at TIRR
2323 S. Shepherd, Suite 1000
Houston, TX 77019
(800) 949-4232l; (713) 520-0232
www.ilru.org
E-mail: ilru@ilru.org

Lighthouse International
111 East 59th Street
New York, NY 10022-1202
(800) 829-0500; (212) 821-9200
www.lighthouse.org
E-mail: info@lighthouse.org
Provides free information on eye-related diseases and can refer individuals to resources in your community. Free catalog on low-vision aides. Includes link to Vision Connection, an interactive resource for latest information on vision; features "Help Near You" function, to find resources in your area.

Medic Alert®
(800) 432-5378
Offers critically important medical facts about the emblem wearer's condition to emergency personnel 24 hours a day.

Microsoft Accessibility Technology for Everyone
www.microsoft.com/enable
A Web site of products, training, and free resources to make technology accessible to everyone.

National Multiple Sclerosis Society
(800) FIGHT-MS (800-344-4867)
www.nationalmssociety.org

National Rehabilitation Information Center for Independence
4200 Forbes Boulevard, Suite 202
Lanham, MD 20706
(800) 346-2742
www.naric.com
E-mail: naricinfo@heitechservices.com
A database of research information about assistive technology and rehabilitation. One-stop shopping for referrals, information, and equipment sources. Fees for some services.

NCM Aftertherapy Catalog
(800) 235-7054

Radio Shack
Carries a variety of alerting devices in stores nationwide.
Check your phonebook for store near you.

Sammons-Preston
Bowling Brook, IL
(800) 323-5547

Sears Home Health Care Catalogue
(800) 326-1750 for customer service
To place an order or find a Sears store near you.

Self-Help for Hard of Hearing People (SHHH)
7910 Woodmont Avenue, Suite 1200
Bethesda, MD 20814
(301) 657-2248; (301) 657-2249 (TTY)
Offers information on coping with hearing loss and on hearing aids.

SpeciaLiving Magazine
www.specialiving.com
Online info and store for accessible housing, special products, such as ramps, bathing systems, urinary devices, lifts.

University of Florida—Project Link
P.O. Box 100164
Gainesville, FL 32610-0164
(877) 770-7303
www.phhp.ufl.edu/ot/projectlink
A nationwide information service, Project Link mails catalogs and brochures from different companies that manufacture assistive devices.

World Institute on Disability
510 16th Street, Suite 100
Oakland, CA 94612
(510) 763-4100; TTY: (510) 208-9496;
Fax: (510) 763-4109
www.wid.org
E-mail: wid@wid.org

Cooling Devices
www.polar-products.com
www.mistymate.com
www.stageoneproductions.com
www.coolbandcity.com

For **medical alarms**, consult the phone book or contact your local hospital's long-term care or senior services division.

If you don't have access to the Internet, ask your local library to help you locate a Web site.

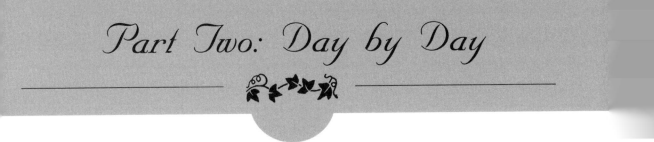

Part Two: Day by Day

Setting Up a Plan of Care

Setting Up a Plan of Care

A plan of care is a daily record of the care and treatment a person needs on a daily basis. The plan helps you and anyone who assists you with caregiving tasks.

A plan of care helps caregivers manage the day-to-day activities of the person in their care—medications, appointments, exercise, etc. This type of written record is also very helpful when respite (relief) care is used.

The plan of care includes the following information:

- *diagnosis*

- *medications*

- *physical limitations of the care receiver*

- *a list of equipment needed*

- *diet*

- *detailed care instructions and comments*

- *services the home health care agency will provide, if using such on agency.*

This information is presented in a certain order so that the process of care is repeated over and over again until it becomes routine. When the plan is kept up to date, it provides a clear record of events that is helpful in solving problems and avoiding them. With a plan you don't have to rely on your memory. It also allows another person to take over respite care or take your place entirely without too much trouble.

Some of the things you may have to watch and record are

- *skin color, warmth, and tone (dryness, firmness, etc.)*

- *pressure areas where bedsores can develop* (📖 *See Activities of Daily Living,* p. 165)

- breathing, temperature, pulse, and blood pressure

- circulation (dark red or blue spots on the legs or feet)

- finger and toenails (any unusual conditions)

- mobility (ability to move around)

- puffiness around the eyes and cheeks, swelling of the hands and ankles

- appetite

- body posture (relaxed, twisted, or stiff)

- bowel and bladder function (unusual changes)

- any changes in MS-related symptoms

Recording the Plan of Care

To record the plan of care, use a loose-leaf notebook. Put the doctor's instructions on the inside front cover (always keep the originals). Include in the notebook the types of forms that appear in the following pages in this chapter. These pages should be three-hole punched.

After using your plan of care for one week, adjust as needed and keep doing so as the person's needs change. Always do what works for you and the person being cared for. Use notes, pictures, or anything else to describe your duties. Also, use black ink, not pencil, to keep a permanent record.

Daily Activities Record (Sample Form)   Day/Date: _____

Morning _____
_____

Afternoon _____
_____

Naps: Time _____ Place _____
Evening _____
_____

Activities	Yes	No	Where/How/When
Walk	❏	❏	_____
TV	❏	❏	_____
Reading	❏	❏	_____
Visitors	❏	❏	_____
Calls to Friends/Relatives	❏	❏	_____
Other _____			

Bedtime Routine	Yes	No	Where/How
Incontinence Pad/Brief	❏	❏	_____
Medication	❏	❏	_____
Special Pillow/Blanket	❏	❏	_____
Music/Radio/TV	❏	❏	_____
Nightlight	❏	❏	_____
Restraints, Calming Techniques	❏	❏	_____
Urinal/Bedpan	❏	❏	_____
Gates at Doors/on Stairs	❏	❏	_____
Oral/Denture Care	❏	❏	_____
Foot Care	❏	❏	_____

Braces ❏   Fungus ❏   Massage ❏   Ingrown Nails ❏   Nail Care ❏

Meals
Help Needed with Meals _____
Meal Times _____
Special Diet _____
Foods to Avoid _____
Special Utensils _____
Snacks _____
Favorite Foods _____
Location of Meals _____

Daily Care Record (Sample Form)   Day/Date: _____

Daily Activities/Limitations:
Walks Alone _____ Stands Alone _____

Bed Position _____

Equipment Used: Walker ❑   Cane ❑   Wheelchair ❑   Brace ❑

How long _____

ROM/Exercises: Upper Body ❑   Lower Body ❑   Goes Outside ❑

Meals: Special Diet   ❑
Breakfast _____

Lunch _____

Dinner _____

Snack _____

Fluids _____

Treatments
Catheter _____

Oxygen _____

Equipment _____

Physical Therapy _____

Special Precautions _____

Resuscitate ❑   Do Not Resuscitate ❑

Personal Care
Bath: ❑ Bed   ❑ Chair

Shower: ❑ Tub   ❑ Bench

Care of Genitals: _____

Nail Care: ❑ Toes   ❑ Fingers

Oral Care: ❑ Brush Teeth   ❑ Floss Teeth   ❑ Dentures

Hair Care: ❑ Shave   ❑ Bed Shampoo   ❑ Bath/Shampoo

Skin Care: ❑ Lotion Upper Body   ❑ Lotion Lower Body   ❑ Powdered

Massage: ❑ Head and Shoulder   ❑ Leg and Foot   ❑ Back

Bowel Movements _____ Voiding _____ Quantity _____

Temperature _____ Blood Pressure _____ Respiration _____

Comments/Attitudes/Conditions _____
_____
_____

Visitors _____

Activities Schedule for Backup Caregiver (Sample Form)

Personal Needs	Yes	No	Where to Find
Cane	☐	☐	_____
Dentures	☐	☐	_____
Glasses	☐	☐	_____
Hearing aid	☐	☐	_____
Walker	☐	☐	_____
Other mobility device	☐	☐	_____

Morning Routine

Breakfast _____ Where Eaten _____

Amount of Help Needed _____

Special Utensils Needed _____

Medications with Meals ☐ _____ Nap ☐ _____

Snack Foods _____ Time of Snack _____

Evening Routine

Dinner _____ Where Eaten _____

Evening Snack _____

Bedtime Routine

Help Needed Undressing ☐ _____ Shower or Bath Needed ☐ _____

Where Clothes Are Stored _____

Where Dentures Are Stored _____

Special Items Needed: _____

Incontinent Pad/Brief ☐ _____ Urinal ☐ _____ Restraints ☐ _____

Special Pillows ☐ _____ Music ☐ _____ Nightlight ☐ _____

Calming Techniques _____

Special Concerns or Equipment

Catheter ☐ _____ Oxygen ☐ _____

Special Precautions _____

Other _____

Resuscitate ☐   **Do Not Resuscitate ☐**

Be on the Alert for:

Gates on Stairs/Locks on Doors _____

Alarms _____

Other _____

Don't be surprised if: _____

Recording and Managing Medications

You must have a careful system for keeping track of medications:

- when medications should be given
- how they should be given
- when they were actually given

The following sample of a weekly medication schedule is a good model to follow. Be sure to fill in the times (A.M. and P.M.) when medications actually were given, and have each caregiver initial them.

Weekly Medication Schedule (Sample Form)

Medication	Date/Time/Initials						
Name, dose, frequency, with food, without food	Sat.	Sun.	Mon.	Tues.	Wed.	Thurs.	Fri.
Disease-Modifying Therapy	Date/Time/Initials						
Name of Drug	Sat.	Sun.	Mon.	Tues.	Wed.	Thurs.	Fri.
Example							
2 mg. Coumadin 1× daily am with food	8:30am	8:00am	9:00am	8:45am	9:00am	8:30am	7:45am
400 mg. folic acid 1× daily am	8:30am	8:00am	9:00am	8:45am	9:00am	8:30am	7:45am
Fruitlax 1 Tbsp. evening only	6pm	6pm	6:30pm	6:45pm	6:15pm	6:30pm	7:00pm
Visine	10am	10am		4pm			

As you finish your own schedule, be sure to record information from the label of each prescription, including the following:

- days of the week when each medicine must be taken
- number of times per day
- time of day
- whether the medicine is to be taken with or without food
- how much water should be taken with the medicine

Also make a note to yourself about—

- any warnings (for example, "Don't take this medicine with alcohol")
- possible side effects (dizziness, confusion, headache, etc.)

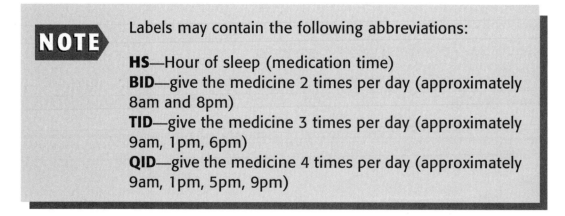

NOTE Labels may contain the following abbreviations:

HS—Hour of sleep (medication time)
BID—give the medicine 2 times per day (approximately 8am and 8pm)
TID—give the medicine 3 times per day (approximately 9am, 1pm, 6pm)
QID—give the medicine 4 times per day (approximately 9am, 1pm, 5pm, 9pm)

Other Cautions

- Never crush drugs without talking to the doctor or pharmacist. If the person in your care has trouble swallowing medication, ask the doctor for another way to give it. (See *Using the Health Care Team Effectively,* p. 23.)

- If the person in your care is going to take the medicine without your help, ask the pharmacist to prepackage dosages or come up with a color code to use when taking several medications.

- Do not store medicine that will be taken internally (swallowed) in the same cabinet with those that will be used externally (lotions, salves, creams, etc.).

- Keep a magnifying glass near the medicine cabinet for reading small print.

- Store most medicine in a cool, dry place—usually not the bathroom.

- Remove the cotton from each bottle so that moisture is not drawn in.

- Flush all medicine not currently being used down the toilet.

- Ask the pharmacist for containers that are not childproof if the childproof ones are too hard to open.

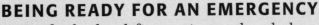

Tip **BEING READY FOR AN EMERGENCY**
Notify the local fire station and ambulance company that a person with disabilities lives at this address. They will have the information on hand and can respond quickly.

Emergency Information

Have this information posted near telephones or on the refrigerator, where it can be used by anyone in the household in case of emergency.

Personal Information (Person in Your Care)

Name _____ Date of Birth _____

Address _____

Phone _____

SS # _____ Supplemental Insurance # _____

Medicaid # _____ Medicare # _____

Current Medications: _____

_____

Exact Location of Do Not Resuscitate Order: _____

Emergency Numbers

Fire _____ Police _____

Ambulance _____ Hospital _____

Doctor _____

Drugstore _____ Open Till _____ Delivers _____

Family Caregiver Work Number _____

Alternate Caregiver _____

Home Health Care Agency _____

Medicare Toll Free Number _____

Insurance _____

Medical Equipment Company _____

Poison Control _____

Friend _____

_____

Neighbor _____ Relative _____

Clergy/Rabbi _____

Transport Number _____ Meals-on-Wheels _____

Shopping Assistance _____

_____

Directions for Driving to the House _____

_____

_____

ℛESOURCES►

Elder Health Program
Peter Lamy Center on Drug Therapy and Aging
University of Maryland at Baltimore, School of Pharmacy
506 West Fayette Street, Room 106
Baltimore, MD 21201
(410) 706-2434; Fax (410) 706-1488
www.pharmacy.umaryland.edu/lamy
Provides free information about older people and medications.

Publication

Review of Regular Medications and Supplements available from National Multiple Sclerosis Society (800) FIGHT-MS (800-344-4867) or www.nationalmssociety.org

If you don't have access to the Internet, ask your local library to help you locate a Web site.

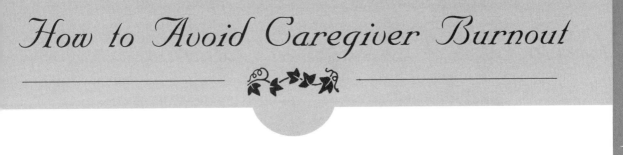

How to Avoid Caregiver Burnout

How to Avoid Caregiver Burnout

*P*roviding emotional support and physical care to someone with MS can be deeply satisfying, but it can be upsetting. Sometimes it is simply more than one person can handle. The strain of balancing a job, a family, more work in the home, and the care of someone with MS may lead you to feel like a martyr or angry and guilty.

One of the biggest mistakes caregivers make is thinking that they can—and should—do everything by themselves. The best way to avoid burnout is to have the practical and emotional support of other people. Sharing concerns with others not only relieves stress, but also can give you a new slant on problems.

Emotional Burdens

You may think you are the only one to face these problems, but you are not alone. Every caregiver faces—

- the need to hide his or her grief

- fear of the future

- worries about money

- having less ability to solve problems

Dependency and Isolation

Fears of dependency and loneliness, or isolation, are common in families of those who are chronically ill. The person with MS can become more and more dependent on the one who is providing care. At the same time, the caregiver needs others for respite and support. Many caregivers are ashamed about needing help, so they don't ask for it. Those caregivers who are able to develop personal and social support have a greater sense of well-being.

> **NOTE** Men who are caregivers face special problems. Often they are not used to doing daily chores around the house. They also lose the emotional support of the spouse who is ill and must now be her support. It is especially important for men to seek out a support system.

Knowing When to Seek Help

"**Why doesn't anyone ask how I am doing?**" It is easy to feel invisible, as if no one can see you. Everyone's attention is on the person with MS, and they don't seem to understand what the caregiver is going through. Many caregivers say that nobody even asks how they're doing. Mental health experts say it's not wise to let feelings of neglect build up. Caregivers need to speak up and tell other people what they need and how they feel.

Support groups, religious or spiritual advisors, or mental health counselors can teach you new and positive ways to express your own need for help.

Seek out professional help when you:

- are using more alcohol than usual to relax

- are using too many prescription medications

- have physical symptoms such as skin rashes, backaches, or a cold or flu that won't go away

- are unable to think clearly or focus

- feel tired and don't want to do anything

- feel keyed up and on edge

Checklist **Dealing with Physical and Emotional Burdens**

✓ Do not allow the person in your care to take unfair advantage of you by being overly demanding.

✓ Live one day at a time.

✓ List priorities, decide what to leave undone, and think of ways to make the work easier.

✓ When doing a long, boring care task, use the time to relax or listen to music.

✓ Find time for regular exercise to increase your energy (even if you only stretch in place).

✓ Focus on getting relaxing sleep rather than more sleep.

✓ Take several short rests in order to get enough sleep.

✓ Set aside time for prayer or reflection.

✓ Practice deep breathing and learn to meditate to empty your mind of all troubles.

✓ Allow your self-esteem to rise because you have discovered hidden skills and talents.

✓ Realize your own limitations and accept them.

✓ Make sure your goals are realistic—you may be unable to do everything you could do before.

✓ Keep your eating habits balanced—do not fall into a toast-and-tea habit.

✓ *Take time for yourself.*

✓ *Treat yourself to a massage.*

✓ *Keep up with outside friends and activities.*

✓ *Spread the word that you would welcome some help, and allow friends to help with respite care.*

✓ *Delegate (assign) jobs to others. Keep a list of tasks you need to have done and assign specific ones when people offer to help.*

✓ *Share your concerns with a friend.*

✓ *Join a support group, or start one (to share ideas and resources).*

✓ *Use respite care when needed.*

✓ *Express yourself openly and honestly with people you feel should be doing more to help.*

✓ *When you visit your own doctor, be sure to explain your caregiving responsibilities, not just your symptoms.*

✓ *Allow yourself to feel your emotions without guilt. They are natural and very human.*

✓ *Unload your anger and frustration by writing it down.*

✓ *Allow yourself to cry and sob.*

✓ *Know that you are providing a very important service to the person in your care.*

- feel sad all the time
- feel intense fear and anxiety
- feel worthless and guilty
- are depressed for two weeks or more
- are having thoughts of suicide
- have become or are thinking about becoming physically violent toward the person you are caring for

When Hostility Builds to the Breaking Point

Anger is a common emotion for caregivers and for the person being cared for. The situation feels—and is—unfair. Both may say hurtful words during a difficult task. Someone may slam a door during a disagreement. Shouting sometimes replaces conversation. Anger and frustration must be addressed and healthy outlets found as a way to let off steam. If they are not, angry situations can become physically or emotionally abusive.

You can control your emotions by letting go of anger and frustration in a safe way.

- Take a walk to cool down.
- Write your thoughts in a journal.
- Go to a private corner and take out your anger on a big pillow.

Where to Find Professional Help or Support Groups

- the community pages of the phone directory
- the local county medical society, which can provide a list of counselors, psychologists, and psychiatrists
- religious service agencies
- community health clinics

- religious and spiritual advisors
- National MS Society
- United Way's "First Call for Help"
- a hospital's social service department
- a newspaper calendar listing of support group meetings
- parish nurses

Ask for help from a counselor who is familiar with the needs of caregivers.

Take Care of the Caregiver

Many caregivers neglect their own physical health. They ignore what is ailing them and don't take steps to avoid getting sick, such as exercising, eating a proper diet, and getting regular medical examinations.

Many caregivers do not get enough sleep at night. If sleep is regularly broken up because the person with MS needs help during the night, talk about the problems with a healthcare professional.

The person with MS needs a healthy caregiver. Both partners need uninterrupted sleep.

How to Let Friends Help You

Outside Activities

Successful caregivers don't give up their own enjoyable activities. Many organizations have respite care programs to provide a break for caregivers. Other family members are often willing—even pleased—to spend time with the person with MS. It may be possible to have respite care on a regular basis. Keep a list of the people you can ask for help once in a while.

If your friends want to know how they can help ease your burden, ask them to:

- telephone and be a good listener as you may voice strong feelings
- offer words of appreciation for your efforts
- share a meal
- help you find useful information about community resources
- show genuine interest
- stop by or send cards, letters, pictures, or humorous newspaper clippings
- share the workload
- help hire a relief caregiver

It helps to remember the saying, "Grant me the serenity to accept the things I cannot change, the courage to change the things I can, and the wisdom to know the difference."

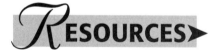

RESOURCES

Caregiver.com
www.caregiver.com
Maintains one of the most visited caregiver sites on the Internet. Publishes Today's Caregiver Magazine. *Provides links to many resources such as government and non-profit agencies.*

Caregiver Survival Resources
www.caregiver911.com
A comprehensive list linking caregiving information and services for general issues and specific chronic illnesses.

Center for Family Caregivers/Tad Publishing Co.
www.caregiving.com or www.familycaregivers.org
Develops and distributes educational materials on caregiving, including a newsletter. Caregiving informational kits are $5 each; please specify new, seasoned, and transitioning caregiver when requesting a kit.

Lotsa Helping Hands
www.lotsahelpinghands.com
Provides a free-of-charge Web service that allows family, friends, neighbors, and colleagues—the community circle of a person with MS—to assist more easily with daily meals, rides, shopping, baby-sitting, and errands that may become a burden during times of medical crisis.

MSWorld
www.msworld.org
MSWorld offers online bulletin boards and chatrooms for people with MS and their family members. There is a board for partners, family members, and friends.

National Alliance for Caregiving
4720 Montgomery Lane, 5th Floor
Bethesda, MD 20184
www.caregiving.org
The Alliance is a non-profit coalition of national organizations focusing on issues of family caregiving.

National Family Caregivers Association
10400 Connecticut Avenue, Suite 500
Kensington, MD 20895
(800) 896-3650
info@thefamilycaregiver.org
www.thefamilycaregiver.org
Free member benefits include Take Care!, *a quarterly newsletter;* The Resourceful Caregiver, *a useful guide to resources; a support hotline and online chat room.*

National Multiple Sclerosis Society
(800) FIGHT-MS (800-344-4867)
www.nationalmssociety.org
Offers a wide variety of programs and services to include self-help groups, for people with MS and their families.

Today's Caregiver Magazine
6365 Taft Street, Suite 3003
Hollywood, FL 33024
(800) 829-2734
www.caregiver.com/magazine
Bimonthly magazine dedicated to caregivers.

Well Spouse Foundation
63 West Main Street, Suite H
Freehold, NJ 07728
(800) 838-0879
info@wellspouse.org
www.wellspouse.org
Publishes Mainstay, *a bimonthly newsletter and provides networking/local support groups.*

Check with your local church or health facility to see if they sponsor **Share the Care** teams.

Publications

Care for the Family Caregiver: A Place to Start, a report prepared by HIP Health Plan of New York and National Alliance for Caregiving. Available at www.caregiving.org

A Guide for Caregivers published by the National MS Society.

Helping Yourself Help Others: A Book for Caregivers, by Rosalynn Carter, with Susan Golant. Random House/ Time Books, 1995.
(800) 733-3000
Plenty of basic information for caregivers.

Love, Honor and Value: A Family Caregiver Speaks Out about the Choices and Challenges of Caregiving, by Suzanne Geffen Mintz

Mainstay: For the Well Spouse of the Chronically Ill by Maggie Strong

Multiple Sclerosis: A Guide for Families by Rosalind C. Kalb, PhD (ed.). Demos Medical Publishing, 2006. 293 pp. $24.95.
Contains chapters on topics ranging from emotional and cognitive issues, to sexuality and intimacy, to life planning.

Positive Caregiver Attitudes by James Sherman, PhD

If you don't have home access to the Internet, ask your local library to help you locate any Web site.

Activities of Daily Living

Activities of Daily Living

Personal Hygiene

As a caregiver, you may find that some of your time each day will be devoted to assisting the person in your care with personal hygiene. This includes bathing, shampooing, oral or mouth care, shaving, and foot care.

The Bed Bath

Bed baths are needed by people who are confined to bed. Baths clean, stimulate, and increase blood flow (circulation) in the skin. However, they can also dry the skin and in some instances cause chapping. Thus, you must decide how often a bed bath is needed. Your decision must be based on the situation of the person in your care. For example, if urinary incontinence (leakage), bowel problems, and heavy perspiration are present, a daily bath may be in order. If not, bathing 2 to 3 times a week might be enough. At bath time, inspect the whole body for pressure sores, swelling, rashes, moles, and other unusual conditions. If baths are given often and the skin is dry, use soap and water one time and lotion and water the next. Cornstarch and powder can cause skin problems in some people. Ask the nurse on your health care team for advice.

> *Tip* **SKIN CARE**
> It is easier to prevent chapping than to heal it, so apply lotion often.

To avoid spreading germs, always wash your own hands before and after giving a bath. At each step, tell the person what you are about to do and ask for his or her help if they are able.

1. Make sure the room is a comfortable temperature and not too warm.

2. Gather supplies—disposable gloves, mild soap, washcloth, washbasin, lotion, comb, electric razor, shampoo—and clean clothes.

3. Use good body mechanics (position)—keep your feet separated, stand firmly, bend your knees, and keep your back in a neutral position. (See p. 274.)

4. Offer the bedpan or urinal.

5. If you have a hospital bed, raise the bed to its highest level and bring the head of the bed to an upright position.

6. Help with oral hygiene—brushing the teeth or cleansing the mouth. (See p. 176.)

7. Test the temperature of the water in the basin with your hand.

8. Remove the person's clothes, the blanket, and the top sheet. Cover the person with a towel or light blanket. Keep all of the body covered during the bed bath, uncovering only one area at a time while washing it.

9. Now have the person lie almost flat.

10. Use one washcloth for soap, one for rinsing, and a dry towel. Have the washcloth very damp, but not dripping.

11. Very gently wash the face first; pat dry.

NOTE Always start washing at the cleanest part and work toward the dirtiest part.

12. Wash the front of the neck; pat dry.

13. Wash the chest, and for females under the breasts; pat dry.

14. Wash the stomach and upper thighs; pat dry.

15. Clean the navel with a little lotion on a cotton swab.

16. Wash upward from wrist to upper arm to increase circulation; pat dry.

17. Wash the hands and between the fingers; check the nails; pat dry.

18. Place a towel under the person's buttocks.

19. Flex (bend) the person's knees.

20. Wash the legs; pat dry.

21. Wash the feet and between the toes and dry well. Use lotion on dry feet. Do not put lotion between toes. This area must be kept dry and clean to prevent fungal infection.

22. Wash the pubic area. If possible, have the person wash his or her own genitals; if not, do it yourself. (Use PeriWash to prevent a buildup of germs.)

23. If a male is not circumcised, draw back the foreskin, rinse, dry, and bring the foreskin down over the head of the penis again. For the female, wash the genitals thoroughly by spreading the external folds. (This must be done at least daily.)

24. Pat the genitals dry.

25. Watch for unusual tenderness, swelling, or hardness in the testicles.

26. Change the bath water.

27. Roll the person away from you.

28. Tuck a towel under the person.

29. Wash the back from the neck to the buttocks.

30. Rinse; dry well.

31. Give a back rub with lotion to improve circulation.

32. Dress the person.

33. Change the bed linens.

34. Trim the toenails if they are long.

> **NOTE** A buildup of earwax may obstruct hearing. Have the ears checked and cleaned by a nurse or doctor twice a year. If the doctor approves, apply a little lotion to the outside of the ears to prevent drying and itching.

The Basin Bath

If the person in your care can be in a chair or wheelchair, you can give a sponge bath at the sink.

1. Make sure the room is warm.

2. Gather supplies—disposable gloves, mild soap, washcloth, washbasin, lotion, comb, electric razor, shampoo—and clean clothes.

3. Use good body mechanics (position)—keep your feet separated, stand firmly, bend your knees, and keep your back in neutral. (See p. 274.)

4. Offer the urinal.

5. Wash the face first.

6. Wash the rest of the upper body.

7. If the person can stand, wash the genitals. If the person is too weak to stand, wash the lower part of the body in the bed.

The Tub Bath

If the person in your care has good mobility and is strong enough to get in and out of the tub, he or she may enjoy a tub bath. Be sure there are grab bars, a bath bench, and a rubber mat so the person doesn't slide. (It may be easier to sit at bench level rather than at the bottom of the tub.) Use the following steps:

1. Make sure the room is a comfortable temperature.

2. Gather supplies—disposable gloves for the caregiver, mild soap, washcloth, lotion, comb, electric razor, shampoo—and clean clothes.

3. Check the water temperature before the person gets in.

4. Guide the person into the tub. Have the person use the grab bars. (Don't let the person grab you and pull you down.)

5. Help the person wash.

6. Empty the tub and then help the person get out.

7. Guide the person to use the grab bars while getting out. OR you can have the person stand up and then sit on the bath bench. Swing first one leg, then the other leg, over the edge of the tub. Help him stand.

8. Put a towel on a chair or the toilet lid and have the person sit there to dry off.

9. Apply lotion to any skin that appears dry.

10. Help the person dress.

Tip

BATHING IN THE TUB

If a bath bench is not used, many people feel more secure if they turn on to their side and then get on their knees before rising from the tub. This is a very helpful way to get out of the tub if the person is unsteady.

The Shower

Before starting, be sure the shower floor is not slippery. Also make sure there are grab bars, a bath bench, and a rubber mat so the person doesn't slide. A removable shower head is also useful.

1. Make sure the room is a comfortable temperature.

2. Explain to the person what you are going to do.

3. Provide a shower stool in case he or she needs to sit.

4. Gather supplies—mild soap, washcloth, washbasin, comb, electric razor, shampoo—and clean clothes.

5. Turn on the cold water and then the hot to prevent burns. Test and adjust the water temperature before the person gets in. Use gentle water pressure.

6. First, spray and clean the less sensitive parts of the body such as the feet.

7. For safety, ask the person to hold the grab bar or to sit on the shower stool.

8. Move the water hose around the person rather than asking the person to move.

9. Assist in washing as needed.

10. Guide the person out of the shower and wrap with a towel. Turn the water off.

11. Apply lotion to skin that appears dry.

12. If necessary, have the person sit on a stool or on the toilet lid.

13. Assist in drying and dressing.

NOTE ▶ Remove from the bathing area all electrical equipment that could get wet.

Nail Care

When providing nail care, you can watch for signs of irritation or infection. This is especially important in a person with diabetes, for whom a small infection can develop into something more serious. Fingernails and toenails can thicken with age, which will make them more difficult to trim.

1. Assemble supplies—soap, basin with water, towel, nailbrush, scissors, nail clippers, file, and lotion.

2. Wash your hands.

3. Wash the hands of the person in your care with soap and water and soak the hands in a basin of warm water for 5 minutes.

4. Gently scrub the nails with the brush to remove trapped dirt.

5. Dry the nails and gently push back the skin around the nails (the cuticle) with the towel.

6. To prevent ingrown nails, cut nails straight across.

7. File gently to smooth the edges.

8. Gently massage the person's hands and feet with lotion.

 NOTE If other members of the household are using the same equipment, clean the nail clippers with alcohol.

Shampooing the Hair

Keeping the hair and scalp clean improves blood flow to the scalp and keeps the hair healthy. Women especially may consider it a special treat to have their hair styled. Shampooing can be done anytime the person in your care is not overly tired. Before a bath may be the most convenient time. Adopt a system that is easiest for you and the person in your care.

SHAMPOOING
To make washing easy, dilute the shampoo in a bottle before pouring it on the hair.

Wet Shampoo

1. Assemble supplies—disposable gloves, comb and brush, shampoo/conditioner, several pitchers of warm water, large basin, washcloth, towels.

2. Have the person sit on a chair or commode.

3. Drape a large towel over the person's shoulders.

4. Gently comb out any knots.

5. Protect the person's ears with cotton.

6. Ask the person to cover his or her eyes with a washcloth and to lean over the sink.

7. Moisten the hair with a wet washcloth or with water poured from a pitcher.

8. Massage a small amount of diluted shampoo into the hair.

9. Remove the shampoo with clean water or a washcloth until the rinse water or cloth runs clear.

10. Use a leave-in conditioner if desired.

11. Towel the hair dry.

12. Remove the cotton from the ears.

13. Comb the hair gently.

14. If desired, use a hair dryer on the cool setting to dry hair, being very careful not to burn the scalp.

OR

1. Cut a round slit at the raised edge of a heavy rubber dish-draining mat so that the end can tuck under the person's neck and the water can drain down into the sink.

2. Seat the person at the kitchen sink with her back to the mat.

3. Place a towel on the person's shoulders and place the rubber dish-draining mat with the round cut against the neck and the smooth edge draining into the sink (beauty salon style).

4. Follow the procedure above, using the sink hose or a pitcher to wash and rinse the hair.

Dry Shampoo

1. Assemble supplies—disposable gloves for the caregiver, comb and brush, waterless shampoo, and towels.

2. Lather the head until all foam disappears.

3. Towel the hair dry and gently comb it.

 You can buy a waterless shampoo from the pharmacy or at a medical supply company.

Wet Shampoo in Bed

1. Assemble supplies—disposable gloves, comb and brush, shampoo/conditioner, several pitchers of warm water, a large basin, plastic sheet, washcloth, towels, and hair dryer.

2. If possible, raise the bed.

3. Help the person lie flat.

4. Protect the bedding with plastic under the head and shoulders.

5. Roll the edges of the plastic inward so the water will run down into a basin placed on a chair next to the head of the bed.

6. Drape a towel over the person's shoulders.

7. Protect the person's ears with cotton.

8. Cover the person's eyes with a washcloth.

9. Moisten the hair with a wet washcloth.

10. Massage a small amount of diluted shampoo into the hair.

11. Remove the shampoo with a wet washcloth until the water runs clear when the cloth is wrung out.

12. Use leave-in conditioner if desired.

13. Towel the hair dry.

14. Remove the cotton from the ears.

15. Comb the hair gently.

16. Use a hair dryer on the cool setting to dry hair, being very careful not to burn the scalp.

EASIER SHAMPOOING
An enema bag attached to an IV pole provides an easy hose for shampooing.

Shaving

Shaving can be done by the person in your care, or you can shave his whiskers with a safety razor or an electric razor. If he wears dentures, make sure they are in his mouth.

1. Assemble supplies—disposable gloves, safety razor, shaving cream, washcloth, towel, lotion.

2. Wash your hands.

3. Adjust the light so that you can clearly see his face but it is not shining in his eyes.

4. Spread a towel under his chin.

5. Soften the beard by wetting the face with a warm, damp washcloth.

6. Apply shaving cream to his face, carefully avoiding the eyes.

7. Hold the skin tight with one hand and using short firm strokes shave in the direction the hair grows.

8. Be careful of sensitive areas.

9. Rinse his skin with a wet washcloth.

10. Pat his face dry with the towel.

11. Apply lotion if the skin appears dry.

 NOTE Never use an electric razor if the person is receiving oxygen.

Oral Care

Oral care includes cleaning the mouth and gums and the teeth or dentures. Always be patient and explain what you are about to do. (The person who refuses to brush his or her teeth can swish and spit out a fluoridated mouthwash rinse.)

1. Gather supplies—disposable gloves, a soft toothbrush, toothpaste or baking soda, warm water in a glass, dental floss, and a bowl.

2. Bring the person to an upright position.

3. If possible, allow the person to clean his or her own teeth. This should be done twice daily and after meals.

4. Be sure the person can spit out water before allowing a sip. Use a water glass for rinsing.

5. If necessary, ask the person to open his or her mouth. Gently brush the front and back teeth up and down.

6. Rinse well by having the person sip water and spit into a bowl.

Special Considerations for People with MS

People with chronic disease need to have healthy teeth and gums. This is necessary to prevent infections that may worsen MS symptoms. Several MS symptoms can prevent a person from getting proper dental care: Fatigue, spasticity (spasms), weakness, tremor (shaking), facial pain (trigeminal neuralgia), and sensory changes (numbness, tingling and or pain) in the hands can all limit a person's ability to brush and floss adequately. The following tips can help overcome these problems.

If the person with MS is capable of performing his or her own dental care:

• Use toothbrushes with built-up handles. Use flossing tools and think about getting an electric toothbrush.

• If standing at the basin is tiring, have the person sit for brushing and flossing.

• Flossing at bedtime is better because it removes bacteria that grows while the person sleeps. If the person is too tired to floss at night, floss in the morning.

• Allow family members or personal assistants to help with tooth brushing.

• Manage tremors by having the person with MS wear a weighted glove while brushing.

Medications used to treat MS can cause dry mouth. Dry mouth can be lessened by:

- sipping water or sugarless drinks often

- avoiding caffeine, tobacco, and alcohol

- keeping a small square of lemon in the mouth or sugarless lemon candies to stimulate the glands that produce saliva

- using a humidifier at night

- using special products available in pharmacies to moisten dry mouth

Denture Cleaning

1. Remove the dentures from the mouth.

2. Run them under water and soak them in cleaner in a denture cup.

3. Rinse the person's mouth with water or mouthwash.

4. Stimulate (massage) the gums with a very soft toothbrush.

5. Return the dentures to the person's mouth.

 NOTE Even a person with dentures should have the soft tissues of the mouth checked regularly by a dentist.

Foot Care

For the comfort and good health of the person in your care:

- Provide properly fitting low-heeled shoes that close with Velcro® or elastic and have nonslip soles. Avoid shoes with heavy soles, running shoes with rubber tips over the toes, and shoes with thick cushioning.

- Provide cotton socks rather than acrylic.

- Trim the person's nails only after a bath when they have softened.

- Use a disposable sponge-tipped toothbrush to clean or dry between the toes.

- Check feet daily for bumps, cuts, and red spots.

Call the doctor or other health care provider if a sore develops on the foot. The person who is diabetic must have special foot care to prevent infections. Serious infections may result in the amputation of a foot.

 NOTE Foot pain can cause a person to lean back on the heels and increases the chance of a fall, so keep toenails trimmed and feet healthy.

Common Leg and Foot Problems and Solutions

Problem	Solution
Foot strain	Visit a podiatrist.
Calluses	Rub lanolin or lotion on the area; do not cut hard skin.
Cramps	Relieve by movement and massage.
Hammer toes and bunions	Wedge a pad between the big toe and the second toe to straighten them; cut holes in the shoe to relieve rubbing.
Leg ulcers (openings in the skin)	Follow the doctor's instructions. Exercise to keep the foot and ankle mobile.
Swollen legs	Follow the doctor's instructions for treatment of the underlying cause.
Varicose veins	Elevate the legs twice a day for 30 minutes. Before lowering the legs, apply an elastic bandage or stocking.

Dressing

Dressing a person with disabilities can be made easier by following a routine. Before you begin, lay the clothes out in the order in which they will be put on.

- Dress the person while he or she is sitting.

- Use adaptive equipment like a button hook and shoehorn. (See *Equipment and Supplies,* p. 130.)

- Use loose clothes that are easy to put on and have elastic waistbands, Velcro® fasteners, and front openings.

- Use bras that open and close in front.

- Use tube socks.

- Dress the weaker side first.

- For a person who is confined to bed, use a gown that closes in the back. This will make it easier when using a bedpan or urinal.

NOTE For a person who is confined to bed, be sure to smooth out all wrinkles in the clothes and bedding to prevent pressure sores.

Bed Making

Making a bed with someone in it will be easier if you follow these steps:

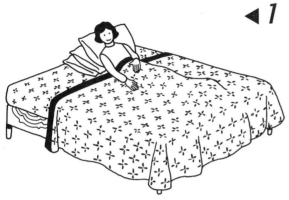

◄ *1*
- The bed has two parts—the side the person is lying on and the side you are making.

- If you have a hospital bed, raise the height of the bed.

- Lower the head and foot of the bed so that it is flat.

Draw sheet

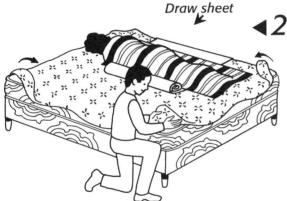

◄ *2*
- Loosen the sheets on all sides.

- Remove the blankets and pillow, leaving only the bottom and top sheets.

- Cover the person with a bath blanket (a flannel sheet or large towel) for modesty and warmth.

- Pull the top sheet out from under the bath blanket.

- Raise the bed rail on the side across from you (the opposite side) so the person cannot fall out of bed. If you don't have a hospital bed, be sure the bed is pushed against the wall.

- Roll the person over to the opposite side of the bed.

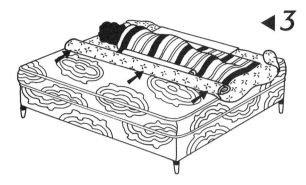

◀3

- Roll all the old bottom sheeting toward the person.

Clean sheet

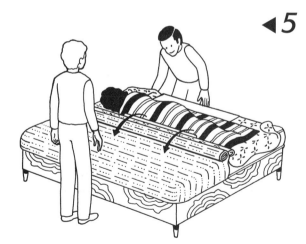

◀4

- Fold the clean sheet, along with other mattress covers, length-wise.

- Place it on the bed with the middle fold running along the center of the mattress right beside the person's body.

◀5

- Unfold the clean sheet and bring enough of it toward you to cover half of the bed.

- Gently lift the mattress and tuck the sheet in.

- Tuck the free edge of the draw sheet under the mattress on your side of the bed.

- Ask the person to roll over the linens in the middle of bed to the clean side.

OR

- Bend as close to the person's body as possible. Place your hand and arm under the person's shoulders and move the person and the bath blanket over the linens in the center of the bed.

- If it is a hospital bed, raise the bed rail on your side and lock it into place.

- Go to the other side and remove all soiled linen. Tuck in all the linen and pull tight on the sheets to remove all wrinkles so they don't rub and irritate the person's skin.

- Change the pillowcase.

- Spread the top sheet over the person and bath blanket.

- Ask the person to hold the sheet while you pull the bath blanket away.

- Tuck the sheet under the mattress at the foot of the bed.

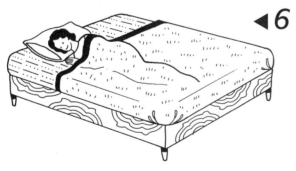

◀6
- Spread a blanket over the top. (The blanket should be up far enough to cover the person's shoulders.)

- Fold the sheet down over the blanket.

- Adjust the person in bed so he or she is comfortable.

Toileting

Always wear disposable gloves when helping with toileting. This prevents the spread of disease. Wash your hands before and after providing care.

Toileting in Bed

When a person is mobile, toileting in bed should not be encouraged.

Toileting in Bed for a Female or for Bowel Movements

1 • Warm the bedpan with warm water. Empty the water into the toilet.

• Powder the bedpan with talcum powder to keep the skin from sticking to it.

• Place a tissue or water in the pan to make cleaning easier. Or use a light spray of vegetable oil in the bedpan, which will make it easier to empty the contents.

• Raise the person's gown.

◀*2* • Ask the person to raise her hips.

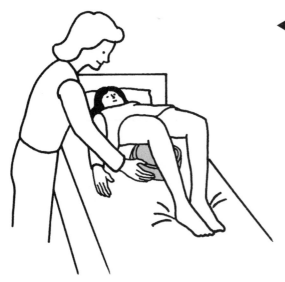

◀3
- If the person cannot raise her hips, turn her on her side and roll the hips back onto the bedpan.

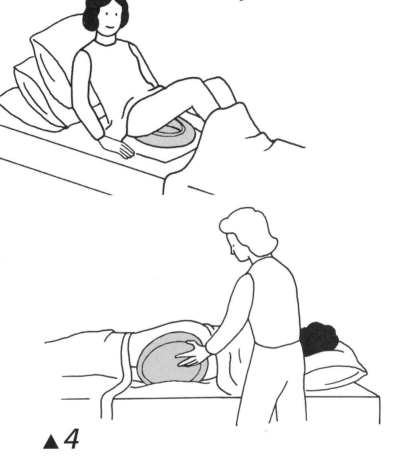

▲4

- If the person cannot do so, clean the anal area with bathroom tissue. Then use a wet tissue to clean the area.

- After the woman has urinated, pour a cup of warm water over her genitals and pat the area dry with a towel.

- Wash the person's hands.

- Remove and empty the bedpan.

- Be sure to wash your hands.

Using a Urinal

1. If the person can't do so himself, place the penis into the urinal as far as possible and hold it in.

2. When the person signals he is finished, remove and empty the urinal.

3. Wash his hands.

4. Wash your own hands.

Using a Commode

A portable commode is helpful for a person with limited mobility. The portable commode (with the pail removed) can be used over the toilet seat and as a shower seat.

Using a Portable Commode

1. Gather the portable commode, toilet tissue, a basin, a cup of water, a washcloth or paper towel, soap, and a towel.

2. Wash your hands.

3. Help the person onto the commode.

4. Offer toilet tissue when the person is finished.

5. Pour a cup of warm water on female genitalia.

6. Pat the area dry with a paper towel.

7. Offer a washcloth so the person can wash his or her hands.

8. Remove the pail from under the seat, empty it, rinse it with clear water, and empty the water into the toilet.

9. Wash your hands.

> **Tip**
>
> **TOILET SAFETY**
> Use Velcro® with tape on the back and attach it to the back of the toilet or commode seat to keep the lid from falling.

Using the Bathroom Toilet

If the mobile person is missing the toilet, get a toilet seat in a color that is different from the floor color. This may help him see the toilet better. If he is failing to cleanse the anal area or failing to wash his hands, use tact to encourage him to do so. This will help prevent the spread of infections.

Catheters

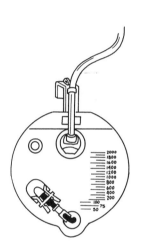

A urinary catheter is a device made from rubber or plastic that drains urine from the body. It is inserted by a nurse through the urethra (a tube that connects the bladder to the outside of the body) into the bladder (an organ that collects urine).

A Foley catheter stays in the bladder and drains into a bag that is attached to a person's leg, the bed, or a chair. When caring for someone with this kind of catheter (called an indwelling catheter), watch for these things:

1. Be sure the tube stays straight and drains properly. Check for kinks in the tubing.

2. Be sure the level of urine in the bag increases.

3. Be sure the drainage bag is always lower than the bladder.

4. Use tape or straps when securing a catheter to someone's inner thigh.

5. In males, an erection is a common effect when a catheter is inserted.

6. Tell the doctor if blood or sediment (matter that settles to the bottom) appears in the tubing or bag.

 NOTE A Foley catheter greatly increases the risk of infection. It is a last resort to manage incontinence (leaking of urine or inability to control bowel movements).

Care of the Person Who Has a Catheter

1. Wash your hands.

2. Put on disposable gloves.

3. Position the person on his or her back.

4. Take care not to pull on the catheter.

5. While holding the catheter, wash the area around it with a washcloth.

6. To avoid infection, wipe toward the anus, not back and forth.

 To prevent foul odors due to the growth of bacteria in the urine drainage bag, put a few drops of hydrogen peroxide in the bag when it is emptied.

Changing a Catheter from Straight Drainage to Leg Bag

1. Gather supplies—disposable gloves, a bed protector, alcohol wipes, and a leg bag with straps.

2. Uncover the end of the catheter and draining tubing; put a towel or other bed protector under this area.

3. Disconnect the drainage tubing from the catheter.

4. Wipe the attachment tube of the leg bag with an alcohol swab and insert it into the catheter.

5. Place the cap attached to the urinary drainage bag over the end of the tubing to keep it clean and prevent urine from leaking out.

6. Secure the tubing to the person's leg.

Condom Catheter

The doctor may prescribe a condom catheter for a male if infections from the indwelling catheter become a chronic problem. The catheter fits over the penis like a condom. Leakage is often a problem with this type of aid. **It is extremely important that a condom catheter not be secured too tightly, which can result in serious injury.** Other products for male incontinence are available that are less constricting, such as Bio Derm's Liberty Pouch, which uses "skin friendly" adhesive.

Incontinence

Incontinence is the leakage of urine or a bowel movement over which the person has no control. It can be a symptom of MS. In addition to bladder management medications, treatments can include bladder training, exercises to strengthen the pelvic floor (Kegel exercises), biofeedback, surgery, electrical muscle stimulator, urinary catheter, prosthetic devices, or external collection devices. Talk to the doctor about the options or treatments for the person in your care.

To Manage Incontinence:

- Avoid alcohol, coffee, spicy foods, and citrus foods. These can irritate the bladder and can increase the need to urinate.

- Give fluids at regular intervals to dilute the urine. This decreases the irritation of the bladder.

- Be sure the person in your care voids (goes to the bathroom) regularly, ideally every 2 to 3 hours. Use an alarm clock to keep track of the time.

- Provide clothing that can be easily removed.

- Keep a bedpan or a portable commode near the person.

- Provide absorbent products (adult diapers) to be worn under clothes.

- Stroke or tap the lower abdomen to cause voiding.

- Keep the skin dry and clean. Urine on the skin can cause pressure sores and infection.

- Your patience and understanding will help the person have confidence and self-respect.

NOTE A precise diagnosis for incontinence must be made in order to come up with an effective treatment plan. If the primary care doctor and neurologist cannot solve the problem, see an experienced urologist familiar with MS.

Urinary Tract Infection

Urinary tract infection may be present if the person has any of the following signs or symptoms:

- blood in the urine
- a burning feeling when voiding
- cloudy urine with sediment (matter that settles to the bottom)
- pain in the lower abdomen or lower back
- fever and chills
- foul-smelling urine
- a frequent, strong urge to void or frequent voiding

Get in touch with the doctor if there is any sign of a urinary tract infection.

Optimal Bowel Function

Maintaining good bowel function can be a challenge, especially in individuals who are unable to get out of bed and get little exercise. For optimal bowel function—

- Set a time for bowel movements every day or every other day. The best time is 20–30 minutes after breakfast.

- Serve fruits, vegetables, and bran.

- Be sure the person in your care drinks 2 quarts (8 glasses) of water daily (or an amount directed by the doctor).

- Provide a chance for daily exercise.

- Use a stool softener or bulk agent if the stools are too hard. When using a bulk laxative, be sure that 6 to 8 glasses of water are taken per day. This will lessen the chance of severe constipation.

- Use glycerin suppositories as needed to help lubricate the bowels for ease of movement.

- Massage the abdomen in a clockwise direction. This can stimulate a bowel movement.

- Avoid laxatives and enemas unless specifically ordered by the doctor or nurse.

Diarrhea

Diarrhea (loose, watery stools) occurs when the intestines push stool along before the water in them can be reabsorbed (taken up) by the body. This condition can be caused by viral stomach flu, antibiotics, or other medications, or stress anxiety.

Diarrhea in people who are immobile is often caused by impaction. This is a blockage formed by hardened stool, with liquid stool passing around it. This must always be taken into consideration, because the usual treatments for diarrhea would be extremely dangerous if the diarrhea is being caused by impaction.

Hemorrhoids

Hemorrhoids are swollen inflamed veins around the anus. They cause tenderness, pain, and bleeding. To treat hemorrhoids, you should do the following:

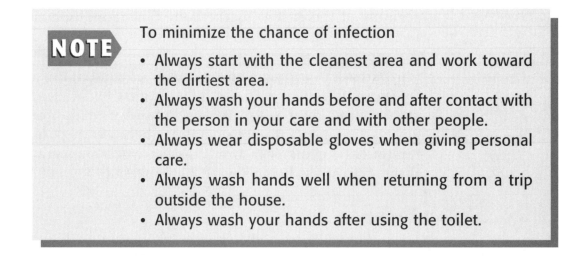

- Be sure to keep anal area clean with premoistened tissues.

- Apply zinc oxide or petroleum jelly to the area.

- Relieve itching by using cold compresses on the anus for 10 minutes several times a day.

- Ask the doctor about suppositories.

Call the Doctor

- if blood from the hemorrhoids is dark red or brown and heavy

- if bleeding continues for more than one week

- if bleeding seems to occur for no reason

Control of Infection in the Home

Common health practices such as frequent hand-washing are necessary to avoid the risk of bacterial, viral, and fungal infections.

NOTE

To minimize the chance of infection
- Always start with the cleanest area and work toward the dirtiest area.
- Always wash your hands before and after contact with the person in your care and with other people.
- Always wear disposable gloves when giving personal care.
- Always wash hands well when returning from a trip outside the house.
- Always wash your hands after using the toilet.

Cleaning Techniques

The following techniques will help cut the chance of infection in the home.

Caregiver Hand-washing

- Hand-washing is the single most effective way to prevent the spread of infection or germs.

- Use bottle-dispensed hand soap.

- If the person in your care has an infection, use antimicrobial soap.

- Rub your hands for at least 30 seconds to produce lots of lather. Do this away from running water so that the lather is not washed away.

- Use a nailbrush on your nails; keep nails trimmed.

- Wash front and back of hands, between fingers, and at least 2 inches up your wrists.

- Repeat the process.

- Dry your hands on a clean towel or a paper towel.

Handling Soiled Laundry

- Do not carry soiled linen close to your body.

- Never shake dirty items or put soiled linens on the floor. They can contaminate (infect) the floor and germs will be spread throughout the house on the soles of shoes.

- Store infected soiled linen in a leak-proof plastic bag and tie it closed.

- Bag soiled laundry in the same place it is used.

- Wash soiled linen separately from other clothes.

- Fill the machine with hot water, add bleach (no more than $1/4$ cup) and detergent. Rinse twice and then dry.

- Clean the washer by running it through a cycle with 1 cup of bleach or other disinfectant to kill germs.

- Use rubber gloves when handling soiled laundry.

- Wash your hands.

 NOTE If urine is highly concentrated due to a bladder infection or dehydration, do not use bleach. The combination of ammonia in the urine and bleach can cause toxic fumes.

Sterilization

If you are sharing equipment with other members of the family, sterilizing will cut down on infection. If you are not sharing equipment, wiping it with a cotton ball soaked in alcohol is adequate.

Wet Heat Sterilization

1. Fill a large pot with water.

2. If sterilizing glass items, put a cloth in the bottom of the pot to prevent breakage.

3. Put items to be sterilized in the pot. These might include syringes, nail trimmers, and scissors.

4. Cover the pot and bring the water to a boil.

5. Boil, covered, for 20 minutes.

6. Leave the items in the pot until ready to use.

 NOTE Cloth can be sterilized by holding a hot iron on it for a few seconds. Never use the microwave oven to disinfect (kill germs) any nonfood items. They can catch fire or explode.

Disposal of Body Fluids

- Wear disposable gloves (recommended for handling all body fluids).

- Flush liquid and solid waste down the toilet.

- Place used dressings and disposable (throwaway) pads in a sturdy plastic bag, tie securely, and place in a sealed container for collection.

Prevention of Odors Caused by Bacteria

Bacteria need moisture, warmth, oxygen, darkness, and nourishment to grow. Some strong odors may be eliminated by

- sprinkling baking soda on the wound dressing

- leaving an open can of finely ground coffee under the bed

- pouring a few drops of mouthwash in commodes and bedpans

- placing cotton balls soaked in mouthwash in the room

- spraying a fine mist of white distilled vinegar mixed with a few drops of eucalyptus or peppermint essential oil

- soaking cotton balls with vanilla extract and placing them in containers that hold on to strong odors

- using electrical and mechanical devices, such as plug-in air fresheners and fans, for removing odor

- buying natural organic room sprays

Skin Care and Prevention of Pressure Sores

Pressure sores (also called decubiti, or bedsores) are blisters or breaks in the skin. They are caused when the body's weight presses blood out of a certain area. The best treatment of pressure sores is prevention. How much time they take to heal depends on advanced they are.

Facts

- The most common areas for sores are the bony areas— tailbone, hips, heels, and elbows.

- Sores can appear when the skin keeps rubbing on a sheet.

- The skin breakdown starts from the inside, works up to the surface, and can happen in just 15 minutes.

- Damage can range from a change in color in unbroken skin to deep wounds down to the muscle or bone.

- For people with light skin in the first stage of a bedsore, the skin color may change to dark purple or red that does not turn pale under fingertip pressure. For people with dark skin, this area may become darker than normal.

- The affected area may feel warmer than the skin around it.

- Pressure sores that are not treated can lead to hospitalization and can require skin grafts.

Prevention

- Check the skin daily. (Bath time is the ideal time to do this.)

- Provide a well-balanced diet, with enough vitamin C, zinc, and protein.

- Keep the skin dry and clean (urine left on the skin can cause sores and infection).

- Keep clothing loose.

- If splints or braces are used, make sure they are adjusted properly.

- Massage the body with light pressure, using equal parts surgical spirit and glycerin. (Ask a nurse or a pharmacist for advice.)

- Turn a person who is unable to get out of bed at least every 2 hours. Change the person's positions. Smooth wrinkles out of sheets.

- Lightly tape foam to bony sections of the body using paper tape, which will not hurt the skin when peeled off.

- Use flannel or 100% cotton sheets to absorb moisture.

- Provide an egg-crate or sheepskin mattress pad for added comfort.

- Rent an electrically operated ripple bed. These beds have sections that can be inflated separately and at different times.

- Avoid using a plastic sheet or a Chux if they cause sweating.

- When the person is sitting, encourage changing the body position every 15 minutes.

- Use foam pads on chair seats to cushion the buttocks.

- Change the type of chair the person sits in; try an open-back garden chair occasionally.

- Provide as much exercise as possible.

Tip

WOUND PREVENTION
If a person tends to scratch or pick at a spot, have the person wear cotton gloves. (Make sure the hands are clean and dry before putting the gloves on.)

When Turning Someone in Bed to Minimize Sores:

1. Explain to the person what you are doing.

2. If possible, raise the bed to its highest position.

3. Lower the head of the bed to a flat position.

4. Loosen the draw sheet at the far side.

5. Stand in proper position as close to the person as possible.

6. Roll the far side of the draw sheet toward you and up close to the person's side.

7. Prop a pillow against the person's back.

8. Flex the person's knees slightly.

9. Place one pillow between the knees and another between the feet.

10. Check any catheter tubing.

Treatment

If you see pressure sores in your daily checking of the skin, you must alert the nurse or the doctor. General guidelines for treatment of these sores are as follows:

- To reduce the chance of infection, wear disposable gloves at all times when providing care.

- Take pressure off sores by changing the person's position often. Use pillows or a foam pad with at least 1 inch of padding to support the body.

- Do not position the person on his or her bony parts.

- Do not let the person lie on pressure sores.

- In bed, change the person's position at least every 2 hours.

- Follow the doctor's or nurse's treatment plan in applying medication to sores and bandaging the areas to protect them while they heal.

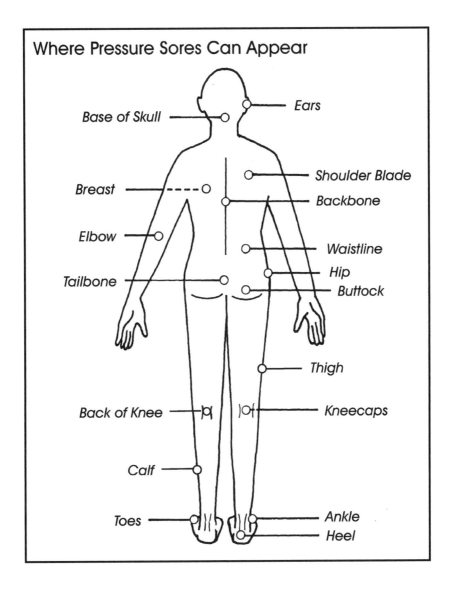

Where Pressure Sores Can Appear

- Base of Skull
- Ears
- Breast
- Shoulder Blade
- Backbone
- Elbow
- Waistline
- Tailbone
- Hip
- Buttock
- Thigh
- Back of Knee
- Kneecaps
- Calf
- Toes
- Ankle
- Heel

Eating

Mealtimes are important because they provide a welcome break in the day. If it is not too distracting for the person in your care, meals can be eaten with the family. It is important that mealtimes be enjoyable so that the person will look forward to eating.

Look for these free or low-cost solutions:

Community meals—local meal programs sponsored by the federal government and open to those over 59 and their spouses. Call the local Area Agency on Aging or Department of Health and Human Resources.

Meals-on-Wheels—hot meals delivered to the home. Call the Visiting Nurse Association.

Food stamps—help based on income that can stretch food dollars. Call the Department of Health and Human Resources or the Area Agency on Aging.

For best results at mealtime:

- Allow 30 to 45 minutes for eating.
- Avoid fussy meal presentation.
- Make sure all items are ready to eat and within reach.
- Provide a comfortable table and chair or other eating arrangement.
- Supply easy-to-hold eating utensils. To avoid cuts, throw out all chipped cups and plates.
- Reduce excess noise such as TV and radio.
- If the person's vision is poor, place the same foods in the same spot on the plate every time.

Feeding Someone in Bed

1. Prop the head with pillows.
2. Provide an over-the-bed table.
3. Do not rush feeding, but maintain a steady pace.
4. Cut the food into bite-size portions.
5. Fill cups only halfway.
6. Let the person hold the cup if he or she wants to. (A terry cloth tennis wristband slipped over the cup may make it easier to hold.)

7. Use available eating aids. (See *Equipment and Supplies,* p. 129.)

8. Keep a moist hand towel to wipe the person's mouth and hands gently. The chains used to hang eyeglasses around the neck can be used to hold a napkin in place.

Tip **FEEDING IN BED**
An adjustable ironing board may be used as an over-the-bed table for activities or eating.

Feeding the Person Who Is Disabled

1. Name the food being offered.

2. If the person plays with food, limit the choices being offered. (Playing with food occurs because a person is confused and unable to make choices.)

3. Check the temperature of the food often.

4. Be gentle with forks and spoons. (A rubber-tipped baby spoon may be helpful.)

5. Feed at a steady pace, alternating food with drink.

6. Remove a spoon from the person's mouth very slowly. If the person clenches the spoon, let go of it and wait for the jaw to relax.

7. Give simple instructions such as "Open your mouth," "Move your tongue," "Now swallow."

8. If the person spits food out, try feeding later.

9. If the person refuses food, provide a drink and return in 10 minutes with the food tray.

10. Between meals, provide a nourishing snack, such as stewed fruit, tapioca pudding, or finger foods.

Boosting Food Intake When the Appetite Is Poor

- Offer more food at the time of day when the person is most hungry or less tired.

- To increase the appeal of food for those with decreased taste and smell, provide strong flavors.

- Use milk or cream instead of water in soups and cooked cereal.

- Add fat by using butter, margarine, or olive oil on foods.

- Add nonfat dry-milk powder to foods like yogurt, mashed potatoes, gravy, and sauces.

- Tell the person to eat with his or her fingers if that is the only way to get the person to eat.

- Offer milk or fruit shakes.

- Offer puréed (finely ground) baby foods.

(📖 See *Diet, Nutrition, and Exercise,* p. 241.)

NOTE If the person in your care needs to swallow three or four times with each bite of food; coughs before, during, or after swallowing; pockets food in the mouth; or senses something caught or sticking in the back of the throat, he or she may have a condition called dysphagia. Difficulty in swallowing is a symptom of MS.

Eating Problems and Solutions

Drooling—Use a straw if possible; help close the mouth with your hand. (However, sometimes the use of a straw can cause choking if liquid touches the back of the mouth too quickly.)

Spitting out food—Ask the doctor if the cause is moodiness or disease.

Too much swallowing or chewing—Coach the person to alternate hot and cold bites.

Difficulty chewing—Change the diet to soft foods.

Difficulty swallowing—Put foods through a blender or food mill; avoid thin liquids and instead serve thick liquids such as milk shakes.

Poor scooping—Use bowls instead of plates.

Difficulty cutting food—Use a small pizza cutter or rolling knife.

Trouble moving food to the back of the mouth—Change the food's thickness and demonstrate how to direct the food to the center of the mouth.

Too dry or too wet mouth—Ask the doctor or the pharmacist if this is a side effect of medications.

Too easily distracted—Pull down the shades and remove the distractions.

 Difficulty in swallowing can cause food or liquids to be taken into the lungs, which can lead to pneumonia. Reduce the chance of food entering the lungs by keeping the person upright for at least 30 minutes after a meal.

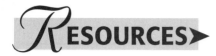
RESOURCES▸

Meeting Life's Challenges
9042 Aspen Grove Lane
Madison, WI 53717
Fax (608) 824-0403
www.meetinglifeschallenges.com
E-mail: help@meetinglifeschallenges.com
Offers a guide called Dressing Tips and Clothing Resources for Making Life Easier, *by Shelley P. Schwarz, a guide to dressing for people with disabilities plus more than 100 resources for custom clothing.*

National Association for Continence (NAFC)
P.O. Box 8310
Spartanburg, SC 29305-8310
(800) 252-3337; (864) 579-7900; Fax (864) 579-7902
www.nafc.org
NAFC is a leading source of education and support to the public about the diagnosis, treatments, and management alternatives for incontinence.

Publications

Bowel Problems: The Basic Facts
Controlling Bladder Problems in Multiple Sclerosis, by Nancy J. Holland, RN, EdD

Sleep Disorders and MS: The Basic Facts

Urinary Dysfunction and MS, by Rosalind C. Kalb, PhD
All of these publications are available by contacting the National Multiple Sclerosis Society: (800) FIGHT-MS (800-344-4867) or www.nationalmssociety.org

If you don't have home access to the Internet, ask your local library to help you locate any Web site.

Therapies

Therapies

The following information is provided for your general knowledge. It IS NOT a substitute for training with professional therapists.

Physical Therapy

Physical therapy is part of the process of relearning how to function after a flare-up or worsening of MS, injury, illness, or period of inactivity. If muscles are not used, they shorten and tighten, making joint motion painful.

What a Physical Therapist Does

A physical therapist treats a person to relieve pain, build up and restore muscle function, and maintain the best possible performance. The therapist does this by using physical means such as active and passive exercise, massage, heat, water, and electricity. Broadly speaking, a physical therapist:

- sets up the goals of treatment with patient and family

- shows how to use special equipment

- instructs in routine daily functions

- teaches safe ways to move

- sets up and teaches an exercise program

 NOTE The American Physical Therapy Association, often located in the state capital, can provide a list of licensed therapists.

What a Physical Therapist Determines

Depending on a person's physical condition, a therapist may work on range-of-motion exercises, correct body positions when resting, devices to help the person in your care, and other simple ways to improve daily functions.

A physical therapist checks things that can affect a person's daily activities—

- the person's attitude toward his situation

- how well he can move his muscles and joints (range of motion)

- his ability to see, smell, hear, and feel

- what he can do on his own and what he needs to learn

- his equipment needs, now and in the future

- what can be improved in the home to make moving around safer and more comfortable

- who can and will help to give support

Range-of-Motion (ROM) Exercises

The purpose of range-of-motion exercises is to relieve pain, maintain normal body alignment (positions), help prevent skin swelling and breakdown, and promote bone formation. A ROM exercise program should be started before deformities develop. Here are some things to do when you are asked to help with exercises at home:

- Communicate what you are doing.

- Use the flats of both hands, not the fingertips, to hold a body part.

- Take each movement only as far as the joint will go into a comfortable stretch. (Mild discomfort is okay, but it should go away quickly.)

Joints Used in ROM

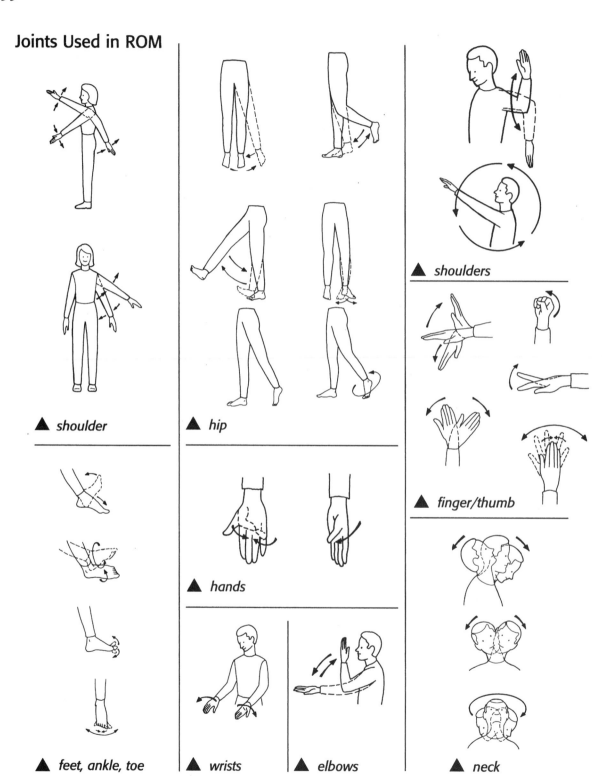

▲ shoulder

▲ hip

▲ shoulders

▲ finger/thumb

▲ feet, ankle, toe

▲ hands

▲ wrists

▲ elbows

▲ neck

- Do each exercise 3 to 5 times.

- Use slow steady movements to help relax muscles and increase joint range.

- If joints are swollen and painful, exercise very gently.

Proper Positions to Use When Resting:

- flat on the back or no more than 30° raised

- prone (lying flat) on the stomach (for up to 20 to 30 minutes only, not for sleeping)

- one-quarter left or right turn onto the back

- three-quarters right or left turn on to the stomach

- aided by special positioning devices (for example, splints for leg, foot, hand, or back support)

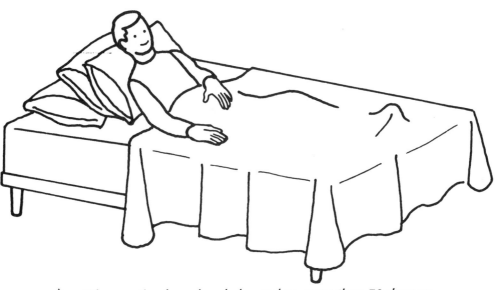

▲ *When resting keep head elevated no more than 30 degrees.*

Occupational Therapy

Occupational therapy is designed to help people regain and build skills that are important for functioning on their own. The occupational therapist will help the person evaluate levels of function.

The occupational therapist will—

- test a person's strength, range of motion, endurance (the ability to continue an activity or effort), and dexterity (skill in using hands) to do everyday tasks that were done easily before an illness or injury happened

- design a program of activities and solutions that ensure the greatest possible independence

- provide training to relearn everyday activities of daily living like eating, grooming, dressing, toileting, bathing, and leisure activities

- decide whether special equipment is needed, such as wheelchairs, feeding devices, transfer equipment, hand and skin devices

- help the person with MS fight tiredness and problems with thinking

Speech Therapy

Speech therapy is the treatment of disorders that involve speaking, hearing, writing, reading, and other communication required for the activities of daily living. Speech therapists also teach people to swallow foods and liquids safely.

A speech therapist or speech pathologist works to—

- strengthen weakened oral muscles through exercises
- teach methods of basic communication

- teach a patient and family how to manage a communication or swallowing disorder

---

Massage Therapy

Massage therapy is an aid to good health because it re-
laxes muscles, increases blood flow, and releases stress.
You can learn to give a simple massage. Never massage
broken skin.

When you give a massage, use only natural oils (olive
or almond). Never use mineral oils or petroleum-based
products like Vaseline.

Back Massage

- Wash your hands with warm water.

- Use warm massage oil or baby powder.

- Expose the back to the top of the buttocks.

- Apply oil to the entire back from shoulders to buttocks
with long firm strokes.

- Use gentle circular motions on each area.

- Dry the back.

Hand Massage

- Wash your hands with warm water.

- Apply warm massage oil or lotion.

- Use short or medium strokes from wrist to fingertips.

- Gently squeeze all sides of the fingers from base to
tip. Use this "milking" motion on the entire hand.

- Lay the person's hand on yours and gently draw your
top hand toward you several times.

- Do not massage portions of the hand that are swollen or red.

TREATING INFLAMMATION

If the finger joints are inflamed, apply ice for the first 24 hours and provide an anti-inflammatory pain reliever, unless the person's physician has not recommended it.

Acupuncture

Acupuncture is one form of treatment in traditional Chinese medicine. It is based on the theory that the body contains a flow of energy. Acupuncture involves stimulating certain locations on the skin by inserting thin, disposable, metallic needles into points along the meridians (or pathways) in the body in order to alter the flow of energy. Similar methods include finger pressure, cupping with small heated cups, and electroacupuncture with electrically stimulated needles.

Acupuncture is a safe treatment for people with MS. It is handled well by most, and may provide relief for some MS-related symptoms, including pain, spasticity (spasm), numbness and tingling, bladder problems, and depression. It is important to remember that acupuncture must be combined with standard medical treatment. Also, the affect of acupuncture on the body's immune system is not clear. People with MS need to discuss this with their doctors before beginning acupuncture.

Horticultural Therapy

Gardening is one of the oldest healing arts. The goal is to improve mental and physical health and the person's spirits.

Advantages of Horticultural Therapy

Horticultural therapy—

- exercises eyes and body
- provides leisure activities when the person can no longer do other activities
- promotes interest and enthusiasm for the future
- provides something to talk about
- encourages a person to walk and bend
- improves confidence
- provides a feeling of being useful
- allows time to daydream
- makes it possible to grow useful house plants or vegetables
- allows a person to be in the sun and enjoy the soothing sounds of nature

To Make Gardening Easier

Make sure that proper body mechanics (positions) are used. Avoid twisting the body, face in the direction of the work being done, and lift using the strength of the upper body and legs. A weightlifter's belt can provide back support.

- Use proper equipment and tools that are right for the person's height and strength.
- Avoid sunburn, chemicals, and hazardous plants.
- Use raised beds to avoid stooping or bending.
- Use perennials, which do not have to be planted every year.
- Use seed tape or mechanical seeders to reduce the need to hold tiny seeds in the hand.

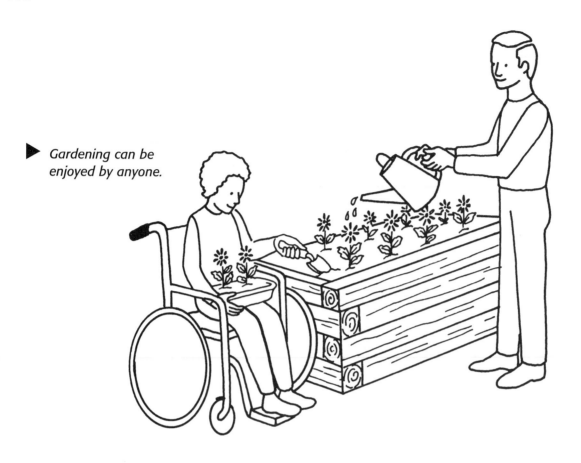

▶ *Gardening can be enjoyed by anyone.*

- Ensure that gardening walkways are 3 feet wide and have nonslip surfaces.

- For those with arthritis, provide gloves that are large enough for foam inserts. The foam eases pain.

- Use tools with cushioned grips.

- Provide foam pads for kneeling or a small stool for sitting.

- To help prevent knee injury, avoid a squatting position. Have the person in your care sit on the ground and move backwards.

- Provide a timer as a reminder to change body position every 20 minutes to avoid repetitive motions.

NOTE If the person in your care is in the garden alone, provide a whistle on a cord worn around the neck or another noise-making device so he or she can call for help.

Aromatherapy

Aromatherapy is a branch of herbal medicine that uses the oils of various plants for medicinal (healing) purposes. These essential oils act to boost energy or calm, aid digestion, and remove toxins (poisons) from the body.

Ways to Use Essential Oils

- with a diffuser—for those with some respiratory conditions

- through outer application—in baths or with massages (2 or 3 drops with almond or olive oil)

- in floral waters—sprayed on skin that is too sensitive to touch

Common Conditions to Treat with Essential Oils

- For insomnia, a room perfumed with lavender or rose in a diffuser is an effective treatment. (A diffuser is a device that creates a mist.)

- For low energy, use geranium and peppermint.

- For relaxation, try cinnamon and chamomile in a diffuser or rubbed on the wrists and temples.

- For pleasant thoughts, try the aroma of ginger, cloves, and allspice.

- To cleanse the respiratory system (lungs, air passages), use eucalyptus in a diffuser.

Essential oils can be expensive but they last a long time. Buy essential oils from a supplier or a health food store. Starter kits with the most widely used selections are available. **Never drink essential oils or use them directly on the skin.**

 NOTE People with medical conditions should consult their health professional before using essential oils.

Pet Therapy

A cat, bird, or dog can bring great joy to people. They provide companionship, relaxation, and a chance to exercise. They also lessen the boredom and fear caused by loneliness.

- Before selecting a dog, check canine-assistant programs in your area. Dogs that were rejected from the program may be ideal for the person in your care.

- Choose a mature dog that is housetrained; do not get a puppy.

- Have a dog or cat neutered or spayed to lessen the chance of roaming.

- Keep up all pet vaccinations.

- Never clean pet cages or feeding dishes in the kitchen sink.

NOTE Be aware that animals carry bacteria and intestinal parasites. Individuals with weakened immune systems should not change the litter box or pick up outside waste and should wash their hands frequently.

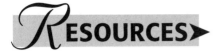ESOURCES➤

Acufinder.com
(760) 630-3600
www.acufinder.com
A referral service that lists state-licensed acupuncturists.

American Academy of Medical Acupuncture
(800) 521-2262
www.medicalacupuncture.org

American Horticultural Therapy Association
3570 E. 12th Ave., Suite 206
Denver, CO 80206
(800) 634-1603; Fax (303) 322-2485
www.ahta.org
Support and education resource for people interested in horticultural therapy.

Charley's Greenhouse & Garden Supply
(800) 322-4707
www.charleysgreenhouse.com
Offers a variety of garden tools that are specially made for those with physical difficulties. Ask for "easy gardening" tools.

Delta Society
875 124th Ave NE, Suite 101
Bellevue, WA 98005
(425) 226-7357; Fax (425) 235-1076
www.deltasociety.org
E-Mail: info@deltasociety.org
Provides information on the human-animal bond and information on how to obtain a service animal.

Gardenscape Tools
(888) 472-3266
www.gardenscapetools.com
Offers a variety of enabling tools.

National Center of Complementary and Alternative Medicine Clearinghouse
(888) 644-6226
www.nccam.nih.gov

National Multiple Sclerosis Society
(800) FIGHT-MS (800-344-4867)
www.nationalmssociety.org

NCM Consumer Products Division
(800) 235-7054
www.ncmedical.com
Sells garden tools that have special handles.

For more information on garden hints, call your local county office of the **Home Extension Service**.

Contact your local **Humane Society** for information about pet therapy.

Publications

Acupuncture and MS: The Basic Facts, by Allen Bowling, MD, PhD, and Thomas Stewart, JD, PA-C

Stretching for People with MS, by Beth E. Gibson, PT

Stretching with a Helper for People with MS, by Beth E. Gibson, PT

Available by contacting the National Multiple Sclerosis Society at (800) FIGHT-MS (800-344-4867).

If you don't have home access to the Internet, ask your local library to help you locate any Web site.

Special Challenges

Special Challenges

*C*ommunication is the ability to speak, understand speech, read, write, and motion with the hands. Nonverbal messages are expressed through silence, body movements, or the look on someone's face. Be aware that words can carry one message, the body another.

Speech Problems

Speech problems in people with MS are caused by lesions in certain parts of the brain responsible for muscle control of the lips, tongue, soft palate, vocal cords, and diaphragm.

- *Dysarthria* is a speech disorder in which speech is slurred or not spoken (articulated) clearly. There may also be a loss of volume control, unnatural emphasis, and slower rate of speech.

- *Dysphonia* is a voice disorder. It involves changes in vocal quality, such as harshness, hoarseness, breathiness, or sounding nasal.

Help is available through a speech/language pathologist (SLP). Medications may be suggested by a physician. Severe speech problems may require the use of a device that makes the voice louder, electronic aids, or computer-assisted communications systems.

Intimacy and MS

Intimacy and sexuality are important to a healthy and contented life. Sexuality does not have to disappear from the lives of couples when one partner has MS. Although people report that their relationships suffer as a result of MS, many people, with or without MS, don't talk easily about their sexuality.

Men and women with MS may want to define sexuality for themselves. This may mean relying more on forms of touching that provide warmth, for example, cuddling, caressing, and massage. Oral and manual stimulation can be highly satisfying alternatives to intercourse. Be romantic, even about everyday activities, so that intimacy grows.

Managing Women's Sexual Problems

Women with MS may have a loss of sex drive, or sensory changes in the genitals, such as vaginal dryness and difficulty or inability to reach orgasm. Medications such as phenytoin and carbamazepine may help with these sensory discomforts. Oral or manual stimulation of the clitoris can help a woman achieve orgasm. Vibrators may also provide stimulation. Water-soluble lubricants are available over the counter to increase vaginal lubrication.

Managing Men's Sexual Problems

The most common problems in men with MS are difficulty or inability to get or hold an erection, decreased genital sensation, and difficulty or inability to ejaculate. Oral medications, such as Viagra, Cialis, Levitra, and injectable medications, such as Papazerine and Alprostadil, are currently used to treat erectile problems, and have been effective in 50% of men with MS. Check with a physician about the latest medications and approaches.

Depression and MS

"Depression" is a term applied to a number of emotional states in MS and is believed to be a symptom of the disease as well as a reaction to it. These states may range from feeling down for a few hours to severe clinical depression that may last for several months. At least half of all people with MS will have serious depression at some point in their disease course.

Symptoms of depression may include sadness or unhappiness that does not go away, tiredness, a change in normal sleep patterns, physical unease, trouble thinking or focusing, feelings of being unworthy or guilt, and thoughts of death or suicide that do not go away.

Depression does not mean a person has a weak character. It should not be considered something shameful that needs to be hidden. It is not something that a person can control or prevent by sheer willpower.

Drug therapy is readily available to treat some of the symptoms of depression. Antidepressants can be prescribed by the primary care physician. Psychotherapy, combined with drug therapy, is often the most effective treatment.

Common Fears of a Person with a Chronic Illness

- loss of self-image
- loss of control over life
- loss of independence and fear of being abandoned
- fear of living alone and being lonely
- fear of death

You can help deal with these powerful emotions by:

- pointing out the person's strengths and focusing on small successes
- restoring areas of control to the person by giving as many choices as possible
- finding new ways for the person to adjust to limitations

- helping the person learn new ways to find meaning in life
- changing your attitude about the person's disability
- being aware that humor is healing and providing large doses of laughter, and providing humorous books, comics, cartoons, television, or movies
- allowing the person to cry upon hearing news of a diagnosis
- allowing for the power of silence
- providing opportunities for peer support and friendship

Seasonal Affective Disorder

Some depression can be brought on by the dark, gloomy days of winter. This type of depression may be treated by sitting in front of full-spectrum lights for 1 hour a day. However, don't trust gadgets that promise miraculous results.

Dealing with Boredom

Boredom can be another problem. It may take all of your and your partner's creativity to fight it. Try the following:

- watching movies
- taking car or bus trips
- listening to music
- taking up hobbies
- going to social events
- playing board games and card games
- attending discussion clubs at the public library and using large print or talking books
- joining activist organizations

- spending time with others in similar difficulties (religious groups, recreation centers, or the YMCA/YWCA)

- being involved in volunteer service organizations

- using a computer and accessing sites on the Internet (which provides an interesting activity and allows the person to communicate with family and friends through e-mail)

Continuing Education

Attending continuing education classes at local colleges or correspondence schools can provide education opportunities, even for those who can't get out of the house. Most schools offer academic and nonacademic classes (for example, boat building, ceramics, and garden design).

To find the program that fits your needs

- Check college programs in your area.

- Check organizations such as museums, botanical gardens, and arts groups.

- Check Internet listings devoted to distance learning.

- Check PBS Adult Service Online, which offers college courses based on their documentaries (see *Resources*).

- Check high-school evening courses.

TUITION DISCOUNTS
Some states encourage older students to attend college by offering tuition discounts at public institutions.

Pain Management

Pain in MS is not uncommon. In one study, 55% of the people studied had "clinically significant pain," at some time during the course of the MS. Almost half (48%) were troubled by chronic pain. Factors such as age when it started, length of time with MS, or degree of disability do not seem to play a part in whether people have pain or not.

There are several types of pain in MS:

One type of **acute pain** in MS is trigeminal neuralgia, or a stabbing pain in the face. This can be treated with medications such as Neurontin or Tegretol. For more advanced cases, there is also a surgical treatment called rhizotomy that severs the nerve roots that carry sensations. Another is called Lhermitte's sign; it is a stabbing, shock-like sensation running from the back of the head down the spine, which is brought on by flexing the neck. Medication is of little use because the pain comes on suddenly. A soft collar to limit neck flexion may be helpful.

Dysesthesia is another kind of pain in which there is burning, aching, or "girdling" around the body. These pains can be treated with Neurontin or with antidepressants such as Elavil. Other treatments involve wearing a pressure stocking or glove, which can change the sensation of pain to one of pressure.

Burning, aching, prickling, or "pins and needles" may be chronic rather than acute. The treatments are the same as for the acute dysesthesias described above.

Chronic back and other musculoskeletal pain are the result of pressure on the body caused by immobility, incorrect use of mobility aids, spasticity, and stress on the body from walking problems. Treatments may include heat, massage, ultrasound, physical therapy, and treatment for spasticity.

Pain Reduction Techniques

The most effective ways to relieve pain are pain medications (analgesics), sleep, immobilization, and distraction. (Heat and cold increase or decrease circulation to the affected area, but should not be used without specific instructions from a doctor.)

To reduce pain, consider:

- distraction through TV, music, or reading aloud
- distraction from a medical procedure by massaging the person's hand
- reduction of stress and promotion of healing through relaxation, meditation, and prayer

 Although good nutrition will not relieve pain, it promotes healing by strengthening the body.

Some types of pain may also be controlled by the following treatments:

- **Acupuncture**—placing needles into designated points of the body
- **Acupressure**—applying pressure and massage at acupuncture points
- **Biofeedback**—monitoring reactions to thoughts by measuring changes in blood pressure, temperature, and body organs
- **Deep breathing**—slow deep breaths taken through the nose and exhaled slowly through pursed lips (relieves pain by increasing oxygen to brain)
- **Opioids**—narcotics provide very strong relief but can be addicting if taken long term
- **Hypnosis**—an altered state of mind that shifts the focus on pain to another idea
- **Meditation**—picturing relief from pain

- **Placebo**—a "sugar" pill that fools the body into thinking it is taking a painkiller and signals pain relief

- **Surgery**—permanent severing (cutting) of nerves to block pain (a serious step that requires careful thought)

- **Topical pain relievers**—creams, rubs, or sprays applied to muscles or joints

- **Transcutaneous nerve stimulator (TNS)**—an electronic device placed over acupuncture points

Cognitive Issues

About 50%–60% of people with MS will have some degree of **cognitive dysfunction**. This means the ability to think, reason, concentrate, or remember have become limited in some way. Of those, 40% will experience moderate problems, and 5% to 10% of persons with MS develop problems that are severe enough to affect everyday activities. There is no relationship between the level of physical disability and degree of cognitive dysfunction.

The cognitive function frequently affected appears to be **memory or recall problems**, especially short-term memory. For example, a person may not be able to remember an important phone number learned that morning. That same person will have no trouble remembering things from the distant past.

Other cognitive changes frequently affected by MS include:

- how quickly a person can process information

- the ability to recognize and draw or assemble things (visual-spatial abilities, which are involved in driving a car and finding one's way around)

- verbal fluency (how easily a person finds and uses words)

227

- multi-tasking
- executive functions, including organizing, planning, prioritizing, and problem solving

Help may be available through the services of these specialists:

- neuropsychologist—who studies behavior, the brain, and the nervous system
- speech pathologist—who studies the nature of speech problems
- occupational therapist—who helps regain and build skills needed for independence

Together, these treatments are referred to as cognitive rehabilitation. More and more people with MS are taking weekly sessions in which they learn a number of ways to help with memory issues, organizational skills, and time management.

Special Management Issues

Swallowing Difficulties

Dysphagia, or difficulty in swallowing, can occur among people with MS. The person may cough after drinking liquids, or choke while eating certain foods, especially those with crumbly textures.

A speech/language pathologist is the professional who diagnoses and treats dysphagia. Treatment usually includes changes in diet, and exercises or stimulation to improve swallowing. In very severe cases that do not respond to these measures, feeding tubes may be inserted directly into the stomach to provide the necessary fluids and nutrition.

Mood Swings

Mood swings or "moodiness" may affect persons with MS and is seen as rapid and generally unpredictable changes in emotions. Family members may complain about frequent bouts of anger or irritability. Mood swings are believed to be a symptom of the disease as well as a reaction to it. Whatever the cause, mood swings can be one of the most challenging aspects of MS from the standpoint of family life. Family counseling may be very important in dealing with this since mood swings are likely to affect everyone in the family. Consult with your health care professional on medications to help with severe mood swings.

Spasticity

Spasticity refers to feelings of stiffness and a wide range of involuntary muscle spasms (sustained muscle contractions or sudden movements). It is one of the more common symptoms of MS. Spasticity may be as mild as the feeling of tightness of muscles or may be so severe as to produce painful, uncontrollable spasms of extremities, usually of the legs. Spasticity may also produce feelings of pain or tightness in and around joints, and can cause low-back pain. Although spasticity can occur in any limb, it is much more common in the legs.

Spasticity may be aggravated by sudden movements or position changes, muscle tightness ("adaptive shortening"), extremes of temperature, humidity, or infections, and can even be triggered by tight clothing.

Treatment Helps Prevent Complications

Left untreated, spasticity can lead to serious complications, including contractures (frozen or immobilized joints) and pressure sores. Because these complications also act as spasticity triggers, they can set off a dangerous increase of symptoms. Treatment of spasticity and muscle tightness by medication and physical and occupational therapy is needed to prevent painful and disabling contractures in the hips, knees, ankles, shoulders, and elbows.

Surgical measures are considered for those rare cases of spasticity that defy all other treatments.

Spasticity Can Provide Some Benefit for People with Significant Weakness

Some degree of spasticity can also provide benefit, particularly for people who experience significant leg weakness. The spasticity gives their legs some rigidity, making it easier for them to stand, transfer, or walk. The goal of treatment for these individuals is to relieve the spasticity sufficiently to ensure comfort and prevent complications, without taking away the rigidity they need to function.

Pseudobulbar Affect

A small percentage of persons with MS experience a more severe form of emotional lability (mood swings) called "pseudobulbar affect" in which there are uncontrollable episodes of laughing and/or crying that are unpredictable and seem to have little or no relationship to actual events or the individual's actual feelings. These changes are thought to result from lesions—damaged areas—in emotional pathways in the brain. It is important for family members and caregivers to know this, and realize that people with MS may not always be able to control their emotions. Several medications have shown benefit in small clinical trials.

Abuse

Abusive behavior is never acceptable. Though tensions can mount in the most loving of families and result in frustration and anger, an emotionally damaging or physically forceful response is *not* okay. When this happens, call for a time-out, and call for help.

Physical abuse usually begins in the process of giving or receiving personal help. For instance, the caregiver might be too rough during dressing or grooming, or the person with MS might scratch a caregiver during a transfer. Once anger and frustration reach this level, abuse by either person may become frequent.

The dangers of physical abuse are easy to see, but emotional abuse is also unhealthy and damaging. Continued shaming, harsh criticism, or controlling behaviors can damage the self-esteem of either person.

Transportation and Travel

Transportation

There are many public and private transportation services that will pick up those who are disabled at their homes. These services rely on vans and paid drivers and run on a schedule to specific locations. Free transportation is available from community volunteer organizations, although most public services charge on a sliding scale (based on what a person can afford).

> **NOTE** Many states ensure transportation to necessary medical care for those who are on Medicaid. Check with your local Medicaid office to see if you qualify.

Community transportation services are provided by

- home health care agencies
- public health departments
- religious organizations
- civic groups
- local American Red Cross chapters

- Area Agency on Aging
- local public transportation companies

Travel

Some group tours and cruise lines cater to travelers who are disabled. Consult the person's doctor before traveling long distances with a person who has a chronic condition.

Tip **TRAVEL PLANNING**
As the primary caregiver, if you are traveling for an extended period, consider investing in a long-distance pager with a toll-free pager number so that you can be reached in case of emergency.

Travel Emergencies

In the event of an emergency abroad, contact American Citizen Services (ACS) in the foreign offices of American consulates and embassies.

American Citizens Services will assist with the following:
- lists of doctors, dentists, hospitals, and clinics
- informing the family if an American becomes ill or injured while traveling
- helping arrange transportation to the United States on a commercial flight (must be paid by the traveler)
- explaining various options and costs for return of remains or burial
- helping locate you, the caregiver, if you are traveling when a family member becomes ill

Travel and Living Wills

If a person becomes disabled with a life-threatening illness while traveling, the medical personnel in foreign countries may not accept the terms of an advance directive. If a person is traveling and has an illness that requires breathing devices or other life-prolonging treatments, it may be impossible to end the treatment without a medical evacuation back to the United States. However, there a few basic steps you can take to ensure that a person's wishes are carried out:

- Take a copy of the living will on the trip. Let any other traveling companions know where it is packed.

- Take health-care-directive documents with you.

- If traveling in the United States, consider signing the form that is used in the state where you might be traveling.

TRAVELING ABROAD

When traveling in tropical countries, use the standard traveler's rule: boil it, peel it, cook it, or forget it!

Travel Discount Guidelines

- The major airlines sell coupon books to those 62 and older.

- Sometimes a caregiver and the traveling companion can get the same discount.

- The companion can use the discount coupon only on the same route and schedule (itinerary) as the caregiver.

- The Canadian Association of Retired Persons and the American Association of Retired Persons (AARP) members can get at least a 10% discount in hotels.

- A Medicare card can be used as identification for travel discounts.

Checklist **Travel for the Person with a Chronic Condition**

✓ Let the person's primary care doctor know of your travel plans.

✓ Take more of the person's medications than needed, along with a list of names and dosages.

✓ If traveling to high-risk areas, check with the doctor to see if a hepatitis A immunization is recommended.

✓ Take a list of all medical conditions.

✓ Use a medical alert identification bracelet for the person in your care.

✓ Take a copy of the person's EKG.

✓ Before taking the trip, read the person's insurance policy to see how "emergency" is defined.

✓ If medical care is needed during the trip, get copies of all bills to support claims for reimbursement.

✓ Check into agreements between the person's health plan and a provider in the area you will visit.

✓ If you anticipate the need for medical care, call ahead to make doctor's appointments in the new location. If the person is covered by an HMO, see if they can help.

✓ Consider buying traveler's insurance. Study the policy terms regarding preexisting conditions. READ THE FINE PRINT.

✓ See if medical equipment is insured for loss or theft.

✓ Consider taking a portable grab bar on the trip.

✓ *If traveling to a foreign country, see if the policy covers having to leave for medical reasons (evacuation).*

✓ *Take the person's health insurance card and toll-free number for travelers.*

✓ *Take copies of the pages in the insurance benefits booklet dealing with emergency care.*

✓ *Carry a card with phone numbers of next-of-kin in case of illness during the trip.*

✓ *Carry a copy of the consular information sheet of the country you are visiting.*

✓ *Write the primary care doctor's number and beeper number on the health insurance card, along with the date of the last tetanus shot.*

✓ *If taking a cruise, ask if a doctor with experience in emergency medicine or family practice will be onboard the ship.*

✓ *If the person in your care has a heart condition, check to make sure your airline carries a defibrillator in the event of cardiac arrest. Most major airlines carry them now.*

✓ *Tell the travel agent or airline that you will require a wheelchair and ask to have your request noted on the ticket.*

✓ *Call ahead to the airport, bus station, or train station to request assistance.*

✓ *If a flight is delayed for more than 4 hours, an airline has a duty to provide a meal that is comparable to the meal offered on the flight, if asked for by the passenger.*

Traveling with Medications

Traveling with MS medications should not stop you from enjoying travel in the United States and abroad. Because many people with MS take drugs by injection, it is a good idea to carry a note from the doctor explaining the need for these drugs and that they are prescription medication. Some tours or cruise lines require a letter from the doctor stating that the person is fit to travel. Here are some tips when traveling with medications:

- Bring enough meds to last your trip plus some extras.

- Pack your meds in a carry-on bag—luggage can stray or become lost.

- Keep all meds in original containers with original prescription labels.

- Carry a used-needle container.

- Make a list of the medications the person takes, and why, with brand and generic names. Make a copy and pack one copy separately.

- Make arrangements for refrigerating the meds.

- Bring the person's insurance ID card, plus instructions for accessing a physician where you are going.

- Bring the doctor's name and contact information, in case of emergency.

> **NOTE** One common fraud is the offer of a "travel agent ID card" to qualify for discounts. The only card accepted as travel agent identification to qualify for discounts is the International Airlines Travel Agent Network (IATAN) ID card.

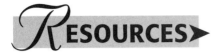

RESOURCES▶

Administration on Aging
www.aoa.dhhs.gov
Information, with links to the Administration on Aging, Social Security Administration, and National Institutes of Health.

American Speech-Language-Hearing Association
10801 Rockville Pike
Rockville, MD 20852
(800) 638-8255; (301) 897-5700 (in Maryland)
www.asha.org
Provides free information on various communication disorders and makes referrals to audiologists and speech pathologists.

Education Index
www.educationindex.com

Healthworld Online
www.healthy.net
Web site with an orientation toward homeopathic, holistic health, and other alternative medicine.

Museums of the USA
www.museumca.org/usa

National Multiple Sclerosis Society
(800) FIGHT-MS (800-344-4867)
www.nationalmssociety.org

PBS Adult Learning Service Online
www.pbs.org/learn/als

Pain Management Resources

American Academy of Medical Acupuncture
www.medicalacupuncture.org
Will provide the names of member acupuncturists who are also medical doctors.

The Worldwide Congress on Pain
http://www.pain.com

Transportation and Travel Resources

Centers for Disease Control and Prevention
(877) FYI-TRIP (394-8747); Fax (888) 232-3299
www.cdc.gov
Provides recommendations on vaccinations and health data for travel to specific countries; also provides information about diseases such as malaria and yellow fever.

Consular Information Program
Bureau of Consular Affairs
State Department
(202) 647-5225 for recorded messages; (202) 647-3000 for automatic fax
www.travel.state.gov
Provides travel advisory information and emergency assistance. Ask for a complete set of Department of State, Bureau of Consular Affairs publications including "Medical Information for Americans Traveling Abroad."

Travel Assistance International
P.O. Box 668
Millersville, MD 21108
(800) 821-2828; (317) 575-2652; Fax (317) 575-2659
www.travelassistance.com
A for-profit company that provides members with worldwide, 24-hour-a-day comprehensive travel services such as on-site emergency medical payments, emergency medical transportation, and assistance with medication replacement.

Publications

Multiple Sclerosis: Understanding the Cognitive Issues, by N. LaRocca and R. Kalb, Demos Medical Publishing, 2006

Multiple Sclerosis: The Questions You Have; the Answers You Need, 3rd edition, Demos Medical Publishing, 2004

The following publications are available by contacting the National Multiple Sclerosis Society at (800) FIGHT-MS (800-344-4867):

Speech and Swallowing: The Basic Facts
MS and Intimacy
Pain: The Basic Facts
Depression and Multiple Sclerosis
Solving Cognitive Problems, by Nick LaRocca, PhD, with Martha King

If you don't have access to the Internet, ask your local library to help you locate a Web site.

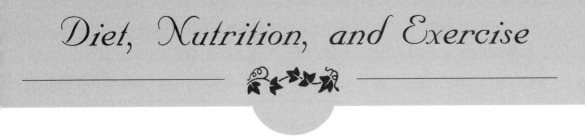

Diet, Nutrition, and Exercise

Diet, Nutrition, and Exercise

Helping Yourself to a Healthier Life

A person's quality of life can often be improved by focusing on those aspects of health that can be changed. Good health has a lot to do with what you do each and every day. Eating right and being physically active are areas in which you can be in control. The lifestyle habits you choose can have a lot to do with feeling good today and staying healthy tomorrow.

A Foundation of Good Nutrition

Bringing good nutrition to the table takes planning, attention, and some imagination. A foundation to healthy eating can be found in the U.S. Department of Agriculture's **MyPyramid**. Making smart choices from each part of the pyramid is the best way to ensure one's body gets the balanced nutrition it needs. Here are some easy tips to make the most of every food group, and get the most from the calories eaten:

- **Focus on fruits.** Select fresh, frozen, canned, or dried over juices for most of your fruit choices.

- **Vary your vegetables.** Choose from a rainbow of colors—dark green, such as broccoli, kale, and spinach; orange, such as carrots, pumpkin, and sweet potatoes; yellow, such as yellow peppers and butternut squash.

- **Make half your grains whole.** When selecting cereals, breads, crackers, or pastas, look to see that the grains listed on the ingredient list are "whole." Whole grains provide a great source of fiber and can help in managing weight and controlling constipation.

- **Keep it lean.** Choose lean meats, fish, and poultry and bake, broil, or grill whenever possible. Try to vary your protein choices and add or substitute beans, peas, lentils, nuts, and seeds to what you eat.

- **Calcium counts.** Include 3 cups of low-fat or fat-free milk, yogurt, or equivalent of low-fat cheeses every day to maintain good bone health. Calcium-fortified foods and beverages can help fill the gap if you don't or can't consume milk.

- **Limit your fat, sugar, and salt.** These "extras" can add up! Check out the nutrition label on foods and look for foods low in saturated and trans fats. Sugars often only provide added calories with little added nutritional value. Choose and prepare foods with little salt or sodium.

Meeting the Challenges of Changing a Diet

Good nutrition is the goal, but food is not just about nutrition. It is about emotions, culture, and being social. What and how we eat is so personal that changing eating habits can be difficult. Special diets and drastic fitness programs sometimes promise the quick fix, or even the cure. Yet, the best advice for people with MS is the same as for everyone: Eat a low-fat diet with a variety of grains, vegetables, and fruits, along with some high-protein foods like meat or dairy products; and balance how many calories you take in with physical activity.

Deciding to change is the first step. But the changes don't have to take place overnight. Start with the easy ones. Then, one by one, add more kinds of vegetables, reduce portion sizes, start eating more low-fat foods.

Here's a checklist for the person with MS:

- Be realistic. Make small changes over time. Small steps can work better than giant leaps.

- Be daring and try new foods.

- Be flexible. Balance food intake with physical activity over several days. Don't focus on just one meal or one day.

- Be sensible and practice not overdoing it.

- Be active and choose activities that you enjoy and that fit into the rest of your life.

Exercise as Part of Life

Physical activity and good nutrition are perfect partners in good health. This winning combination finds a balance between what one eats and one's daily activities. Together they help in managing weight and providing energy. Physical activity not only burns calories, but it can also help the person in your care by doing the following:

- Make the most of muscle strength, or even build strength, depending on the program.

- Slowly increase the ability to do more for longer periods of time.

- Increase range of motion and joint flexibility (the ability to move easily).

- Strengthen the heart.

- Decrease feelings of fatigue.

- Decrease symptoms of depression.

- Maintain regular bowel and bladder functions.

- Cut down on the risk of skin breakdown and irritation.

- Protect weight-bearing bone mass (spine, hips, legs).

Aerobic activities raise the heart rate and breathing, and promote cardiovascular (heart and lung) fitness. Other activities develop strength and flexibility. For example, lifting weights develops strength and can help maintain good bone health. Activities like yoga and gentle stretching can improve flexibility.

Some key points to remember:

- You and the person in your care should talk with the doctor about exercise, target weight, and special needs. If possible, get a referral to a physical therapist to help begin the program.

- An exercise program needs to match the abilities and limitations of the individual. A physical therapist who has worked with people with MS can design a well-balanced exercise program. With some changes, people at all levels of disability can enjoy the benefits of exercise.

- The person in your care should commit to doing what he or she can do on a consistent basis. Choosing activities you both enjoy will help you stick to your fitness plan.

- Start slowly. If the person in your care hasn't been active, begin at a low level of intensity for short periods. Alternate brief periods of exercise with periods of rest until the person in your care begins to build up endurance. Gradually increase how hard you are exercising and the length of time you are doing it.

- Keep your cool. Working out too hard and being overheated can increase fatigue and other MS symptoms for a short time. Drink plenty of fluids before, during, and after the activity. Try exercising in cool water or in an air-conditioned space. For some, using a cooling vest or neck wrap helps keep the core body temperature at the proper level.

- Join a group! Exercising with others may give you the motivation and support to keep going.

Special Needs and Considerations

Good nutrition is necessary for everyone, but sometimes things can get in the way of eating right. For people with MS, it's important to know how MS symptoms or medications can affect nutritional well-being. Ask the nurse, doctor, or pharmacist if any of the medications the person in your care is taking have possible side effects that can interfere with appetite or affect the absorption of important vitamins and minerals.

Managing fatigue is a major issue in MS. Although MS-related fatigue can decrease activity and interest in eating and food preparation, not eating well can actually *contribute* to fatigue. Food is the fuel that one's body needs to function, so missing meals can compromise energy levels. If fatigue is interfering with activities, discuss the problem with a health care professional.

Here are some tips to ensure that the person in your care gets the nutrition he or she needs when fatigue becomes a problem.

- The thought of three big meals may be too much for the person. In fact, five to six smaller mini-meals throughout the day may be easier to manage and help keep energy levels high. Keep the fridge and pantry filled with items that provide the nutrition the person in your care needs for good health and watch those that provide little to the diet except calories. Some healthful choices can include reduced-fat cheese sticks, nuts and nut butter, fresh or dried fruit, hard-boiled eggs, low-fat yogurt or cottage cheese, bagged salads, and cut raw vegetables.

- Keep meal preparation simple. Focus on one part of the meal, like the main dish and rely on quick-cooking grains, easy-to-heat veggies and a whole-grain roll for side dishes. Save energy by collecting all the ingredients and cooking utensils first and sit down at the counter or table to put it all together.

- When you cook, try to make more than is needed for one meal. Store or freeze the rest in oven- or microwave-ready containers for quick reheating.

- Make the most of the freezer. Stock up on low-fat dinners that can be quickly reheated.

- Save menus from places that deliver healthful meals.

Changes in mobility. Some MS symptoms can reduce one's ability to get around (mobility) or do physical activity. If eating habits remain the same while activity drops off, *weight gain* can result. Added weight can increase fatigue, further limit mobility, put a strain on the respiratory and circulatory systems (lungs, heart, blood, blood vessels), and increase the risk of other chronic illnesses. Ask a registered dietitian to recommend an ideal weight and reasonable daily calorie intake to maintain that weight. To get weight under control, pair exercise with healthy eating.

Additionally, inadequate physical activity, lack of weight-bearing exercise, and an increasingly sedentary lifestyle can result from changes in mobility that can contribute to the risk of developing *osteoporosis*—a condition where bones can become thin and fragile. While building strong bones started early in childhood, keeping them healthy as we grow older requires attention and care. Good nutrition—particularly daily sources of calcium—is important for maintaining bone health.

- Choose nonfat or low-fat dairy products often.

- Eat any type of fish with edible bones, such as canned salmon or sardines.

- Choose dark-green vegetables like kale, broccoli, turnip greens, and mustard greens. The calcium in these veggies is better absorbed than the calcium found in spinach, rhubarb, beet greens, and almonds.

- Calcium-fortified tofu, soymilk, orange juice, breads, and cereals are excellent staples. Check the food labels to see just how much calcium has been added.

- Vitamin D also plays an important role in bone health by helping with the calcium absorption. Our bodies can make vitamin D with just 15–20 minutes of skin exposure to the sun each day. Vitamin D can also be found fortified in foods that contain calcium. Be careful with supplementation because vitamin D is stored in the body and can be toxic in relatively low amounts (>2,000 i.u./day)

Eating and emotions. Depression can affect people's appetite in different ways. Many people turn to certain foods for comfort when they are depressed. These may be old favorites from childhood—a scoop of mashed potatoes, macaroni and cheese, a bowl of rice pudding. The danger is in overdoing it. These foods are often high in fat, sugar, and calories that can easily add up. On the other hand, some people lose their appetite when they are depressed. Eating with others can help you and the person in your care stay connected. Remember also that being physically active can help decrease the symptoms of depression.

Bladder problems are another issue. Quite often, fear of having to go to the bathroom frequently or loss of bladder control causes a person to limit fluids. This can cause other problems such as dehydration, dry mouth, difficulty swallowing, loss of appetite, and constipation. Find ways to fit in fluids.

- Take water breaks during the day.

- Have a beverage with meals.

- "Water down" your meals and snacks.

- Take a drink when you pass a water fountain.

- Travel with your own personal supply of bottled water.

Bowel management often involves preventing constipation. Fiber counts . . . add it up. Fiber is found in cereal, grains, nuts, seeds, vegetables, and fruit. It is not completely digested (broken down) or absorbed (taken in) by the body. A diet rich in fiber (about 25 to 30 grams each day) along with adequate fluid intake and physical activity can help promote good bowel function. Fiber can also provide a sense of fullness, which helps in managing how much one eats.

Chewing and swallowing can be a problem for people with MS. Here are some food tips that will help:

- Thicker drinks are easier to swallow. Such drinks may include milk shakes, fruit sauces, sherbets and puddings.

- Foods that crumble easily can cause choking. Avoid giving chips, crackers, toast, and cakes to the person in your care.

- Soft foods need less chewing. Serve eat mashed or baked potatoes, cooked vegetables, and stewed fruits.

- Serve small, frequent meals so that the person doesn't become tired from chewing and swallowing.

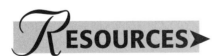

RESOURCES

American Dietetic Association
(800) 366-1655
Call weekdays 10:00 a.m. to 5:00 p.m. EST to locate a registered dietitian in your area.

Area Agency on Aging or the **Cooperative Extension Service**
Your local office offers free counseling by a registered dietitian.

Meals-on-Wheels
Can provide nutritious meals delivered to the home.

MyPyramid
www.mypyramid.gov
This replaces the old Food Guide Pyramid. It is a very interactive site to help people make healthy choices consistent with the 2005 Dietary Guidelines for Americans.

Adaptive Sports

Adventures Within, Inc.
1250 South Ogden Street
Denver, CO 80210
(303) 744-8313
www.adventureswithin.org
E-mail: adwithin@aol.com
This nonprofit organization specializes in providing safe Outward Bound West adventures tailored to the many different abilities and skill levels of people with MS.

The Heuga Center
27 Main Street, Suite 303
Edwards, CO 81632
(800) 367-3101
www.heuga.org
Nonprofit organization that runs a variety of helpful wellness programs for people with MS.

The National Sports Center for the Disabled (NSCD)
P.O. Box 1290
Winter Park, CO 80482
(970) 726-1540
www.nscd.org
E-mail: info@nscd.org
NSCD is a nonprofit corporation that offers winter and summer recreation. Winter sports include snow skiing, snowshoeing, and cross-country skiing. Summer recreation activities include fishing, hiking, rock climbing, whitewater rafting, camping, mountain biking, sailing, therapeutic horseback riding, and a baseball camp.

Publications

A Modification of the Rules of Golf for Golfers with Disabilities
United States Golf Association
P.O. Box 708
Far Hills, NJ 07931-0708
(908) 234-2300.
www.usga.org/playing/rules/golfers_with_disabilities.
html
Online publication contains permissible modifications to the rules of golf for players who are disabled.

Food for Thought: MS and Nutrition by Denise M. Nowack, RD, and Jane Sarnoff
Exercise as Part of Everyday Life by Mary Harmon
Vitamins, Minerals and Herbs in MS: An Introduction by Allen Bowling, PhD, MD and Thomas Stewart, JD, PA-C
All are available from the National Multiple Sclerosis Society at (800) FIGHT-MS (800-344-4867).

If you don't have access to the Internet, ask your local library to help you locate a Web site.

Emergencies

Emergencies

$\mathcal{E}$mergency situations are common when caring for a person with chronic illness. Many injuries can be avoided through preventive measures (See **Preparing the Home,** p. 97). When a crisis does occur, use common sense, stay calm, and realize that you can help.

 NOTE Make sure 911 is posted on your phone or ideally is on speed-dial. Keep written driving instructions near the phone for how to get to your house. If you have a speakerphone, use the speaker when talking to the dispatcher. This way, you can follow the dispatcher's instructions while attending to the emergency.

When to Call for an Ambulance

Call for an ambulance if a person—

- becomes unconscious
- has chest pain or pressure
- has trouble breathing
- has no signs of respiration (is conscious but not able to respond)
- is bleeding severely
- is vomiting blood or is bleeding from the rectum
- has fallen and may have broken bones
- has had a seizure

- has a severe headache and slurred speech
- has pressure or severe pain in the abdomen that does not go away

OR

- if moving the person could cause further injury
- if traffic or distance would cause a life-threatening delay in getting to the hospital
- if the person is too heavy for you to lift or help

Ambulance service is expensive and may not be covered by insurance. Use it when you believe there is an emergency.

In an emergency:

Step 1: Call 911.
Step 2: Care for the victim.

Also call 911 for emergencies involving fire, explosion, poisonous gas, fallen electrical wires, or other life-threatening situations.

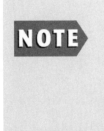

NOTE If the person in your care has signed a Do Not Resuscitate (DNR) order, have it available to show the paramedics. Otherwise, they are required to initiate resuscitation (reviving the person). The order must go with the patient. The Do Not Resuscitate order *must* be with the patient at all times.

In the Emergency Room

Be sure you understand the instructions for care before leaving the emergency room. Call the patient's personal doctor as soon as possible and let him or her know about the emergency room care.

Bring to the emergency room—

- insurance policy numbers
- a list of medical problems
- a list of medications currently being taken
- the personal physician's name and phone number
- the name and number of a relative or friend of the person in your care

We strongly suggest that you take a course in CPR from your local American Red Cross, hospital, or other agency.

Choking (Adult)

Prevention

- Avoid serving excessive alcohol.
- Make sure the person in your care has a good set of dentures to chew food properly.
- Cut the food into small pieces.
- For a person who has had a stroke, use thickening powder in liquids as directed.
- Do not encourage the person to talk while eating.
- Do not make the person laugh while eating.
- Learn the Heimlich maneuver in CPR class.

Bleeding

If someone is bleeding heavily, protect yourself with rubber gloves, plastic wrap, or layers of cloth. Then—

1. Apply direct pressure over the wound with a clean cloth.

2. Apply another clean cloth on top of the blood-soaked cloth, keeping the pressure firm.

3. If no bones are broken, elevate (raise) the injured limb to decrease blood flow.

4. Call 911 for an ambulance.

5. Apply a bandage snugly over the dressing.

6. Wash your hands with soap and water as soon as possible after providing care.

7. Avoid contact with blood-soaked objects.

Shock

Shock may be associated with heavy bleeding, hives, shortness of breath, dizziness, swelling, thirst, and chest pain. The signs of shock are:

- restlessness and irritability

- confusion, altered consciousness

- pale, cool, moist skin

- rapid breathing and weakness

If these signs are present—

1. Have the person lie down.

2. Control any bleeding.

3. Keep the person warm.

4. Elevate the legs about 12 to 14 inches unless the neck or back has been injured.

5. Do not give the person anything to eat or drink.

6. Call 911.

Burns

1. Stop the burning process by pouring large amounts of cold water over the burn.

2. Do *not* remove clothing stuck to the burned area.

3. Cover the burn with a dry, clean covering.

4. Keep the person warm.

5. For *chemical burns to the eyes,* flush the eyes with large amounts of cool running water from the faucet or shower.

OR

Immerse the person's face in water and have the person open and close his eyes.

6. Call 911 for transport to hospital.

Chest Pain

Any chest pain that lasts more than a few minutes is related to the heart until proven otherwise. Call 911 immediately. Don't wait to see if it goes away. Danger signs include—

- pain radiating from the chest down the arms, up the neck to the jaw, and into the back

- crushing, squeezing chest pain or heavy pressure in the chest

- shortness of breath, sweating, nausea and vomiting, weakness

- bluish, pale skin

- skin that is moist

- excessive perspiration

If the person is not breathing, begin Rescue Breathing, and check for signs of respiration (breathing, coughing, moving).

If there are no signs of circulation, begin CPR.

Falls and Related Injuries

Preventive measures include—

- staying in when it is rainy or icy outside

- having regular vision screening check-ups for correct eyeglasses

- using separate reading glasses and other regular glasses if bifocals make it difficult to see the floor

- being cautious when walking on wet floors

- wearing good foot support when walking

- being aware that new shoes are slippery and crepe-soled shoes can cause the toe to catch

- having foot pain problems corrected

- keeping toenails trimmed and feet healthy for good balance

A good way to tell if a part of the body has been injured in a fall is to compare it with an uninjured part. For example, compare the injured leg with the uninjured leg. Do they look and feel the same? Do they move the same way?

When you suspect a *broken bone,* follow these steps:

- If the person *cannot* move or use the injured limb, keep it from moving. Do not straighten a deformed arm or leg. Splint an injury in the position you find it.

- Support the injured part above and below the site of the injury by using folded towels, blankets, pillows, or magazines.

- If the person is face down, roll him over with the "logrolling" technique (see illustration). If you have no one to help you and the victim is breathing adequately, leave the person in the same position.

- If the person does not complain of neck pain but is feeling sick to the stomach, turn the person on one side.

- If the person complains of neck pain, keep his neck steady by putting a few pillows on either side of his head. Keep the head flat.

- Place a piece of cloth on the injury site and apply ice over the cloth.

- Keep the person warm with a blanket and make the person as comfortable as possible.

- Make a splint with cardboard or rolled-up newspaper.

▶ *Log rolling technique—Turning a person safely from the stomach onto the back.*

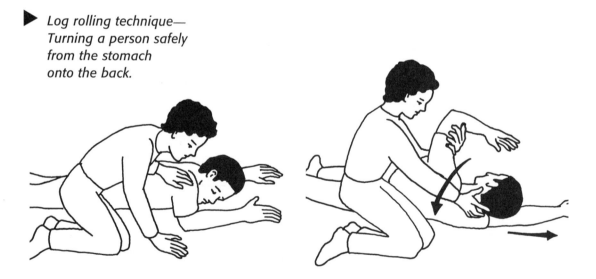

> **NOTE** If an arm or shoulder is splinted, you might consider transporting the person by car. For neck, hip, thigh, back, and pelvic injuries, use an ambulance because the person needs to lie flat.

Fainting

Fainting can be caused by—

- a heart attack
- medications
- low blood sugar
- standing up quickly
- straining to have a bowel movement
- dehydration

To some extent, fainting can be prevented.

- Ask the doctor if medications that do not cause fainting can be prescribed.
- Monitor blood sugar levels.
- Avoid constipation.
- Do not let the person stand up or sit up too rapidly.

If a fainting spell occurs:

1. Do not try to place the person in a sitting position. Instead, immediately lay him down flat.
2. Check the person's airway, breathing, and pulse.
3. Turn the person on his side.
4. Elevate the legs.
5. Cover him with a blanket if the room or floor is cold.

6. Do not give fluids.

7. Use CPR if necessary.

Hypothermia

Hypothermia occurs when a person's body temperature falls below normal (around 98.6°F). Conditions that may alter the person's body response to cold are:

- hypothyroidism (slow thyroid activity)
- arthritis
- dizziness and resulting falls
- excessive alcohol
- stroke
- head injuries
- medications that cause poor body-temperature regulation

To prevent hypothermia—

- Keep the house temperature no lower than 65°F (70°F if the person is ill).
- Have him wear warm clothes, and place wool leg warmers on his arms and legs for extra warmth.
- Use warm blankets when the person is in bed.
- Have him wear a warm hat outside or a knit hat indoors to keep from losing body heat.
- Provide a balanced diet.
- Provide exercise of some sort.

Signs of hypothermia include impaired judgment, shivering, cold pale skin, slow breathing and pulse, weakness, drowsiness, and confusion. If these signs are present, do the following:

1. Wrap the person in blankets, notify the doctor, give warm fluids, and increase room temperature.

2. Avoid rubbing the person's skin.

3. Do not rewarm the person rapidly. Use a heater on low or warm hot-water bottles on the chest and abdomen.

4. Do not give the person alcohol.

5. Be alert to signs of a heart attack (📖 See p. 258).

Heat Stroke

Some medications can increase the likelihood of heat stroke. To prevent heat stroke—

*   Ask the doctor if the medicine the person is taking can increase the risk of heat stroke.

*   Use clothing made of breathable lightweight fabrics.

*   Use a fan, damp compresses, or an air conditioner.

*   Have the person drink 6–8 glasses of water even if not feeling thirsty.

*   Avoid alcohol, caffeine, and smoking because they speed dehydration.

*   Avoid activity during the hottest part of the day.

Signs of heat stroke include headache, nausea, and sudden dizziness. Consult the doctor immediately to determine whether it is a serious condition.

Poisons

If you suspect poisoning, immediately take these steps:

1. Determine *what* was swallowed, *how much,* and at *what time.*

2. Check the person's airway, breathing, and pulse.

3. Contact the nearest Poison Control Center or call 911 for treatment; have the container of the suspected poison at hand.

4. Follow up with the doctor.

5. If necessary, start CPR.

6. If necessary, call 911.

Seizures

A seizure usually lasts from 1 to 5 minutes. If it lasts longer than you are comfortable with or more than 7 minutes, call 911 for an ambulance.

1. Remove all objects that might cause the person to injure himself.

2. Place pillows and blankets around him to protect him.

3. Do *not* hold or restrain the person.

4. Do *not* place anything in the person's mouth.

5. Always check for *breathing* and *signs of circulation* after the seizure stops.

6. If the person is not breathing, administer Rescue Breathing and check often for signs of respiration (breathing, coughing, moving).

7. Call 911.

8. If there are *no signs of respiration*, start CPR.

9. Continue CPR until help arrives.

Stroke

Strokes occur when the blood flow to the brain is interrupted by a clogged or burst blood vessel. Strokes cannot always be prevented, but the chances of their occurring can be lessened through—

- a balanced diet

- avoidance of stress

- periodic checkups

- regular exercise

- regular use of a prescribed blood pressure medicine

Suspect a stroke when the person in your care—

- has a sudden and severe headache

- does not respond to simple statements

- has a seizure

- is suddenly incontinent (unable to control bladder and bowel)

- has paralysis in (cannot move) an arm or leg

- cannot grip equally with both hands

- appears droopy on one side of the face

- has slurred speech or blurred vision

- is confused

- has an unsteady gait

- has trouble swallowing

- has loss of balance or coordination when combined with one of the other signs

The chance of recovery from a stroke is greatly increased if the person has immediate help.

1. Keep the person in the position you found him in.

2. Reassure him and keep him calm.

3. If he has trouble breathing, open his airway, tilt his head, and lift his chin.

4. Check for signs of circulation (breathing, coughing, moving).

5. If the person is not breathing, give 2 Rescue Breaths.

6. If breathing resumes, place the person on one side to prevent choking. This also helps keep the tongue out of the airway.

7. Call 911. Get the person to medical care as soon as possible.

When MS Requires a Trip to the ER

You will learn over time which symptoms will pass and which need the attention of a physician or other health professional. Every symptom is not necessarily an emergency.

However, if you or the person in your care ever thinks there is an emergency in regard to MS symptoms or other chronic conditions, call the doctor's office immediately. It is important to say that you need an appointment right away. If you can't be scheduled, be sure to ask for a referral to the closest emergency room. Many insurance companies require a larger copayment for emergency room visits if your physician does not send you there.

Deciding what is and is not an emergency is up to your physician. It helps to know that the main emergencies in MS are infections, high fevers, falling and breaking a bone, or a sudden or noticeable change in symptoms.

Checklist **Home First Aid Kit**

Buy or make a home first-aid kit. Note on the box the date when the item was purchased. Check and re-plenish your supplies at least once a year. These should include the following:

✓ antibiotic ointment

✓ Band-Aids®

✓ disinfectant for cleaning wounds

✓ disposable gloves

✓ emergency telephone numbers

✓ eye pads

✓ instant ice packs

✓ list of current medications

✓ rolled gauze and elastic bandages

✓ scissors

✓ sterile gauze bandages (nonstick 4"×4")

✓ thermometer

✓ tongue depressors

✓ 3-ounce rubber bulb to rinse out wounds

✓ triangle bandage

✓ tweezers and needle

Body Mechanics—Positioning, Moving, and Transfers

Body Mechanics—Positioning, Moving, and Transfers

Body Mechanics for the Caregiver

Body mechanics involves standing and moving one's body so as to prevent injury, avoid fatigue, and make the best use of strength. When you learn how to control and balance your own body, you can safely control and move another person. Back injuries to nursing home aides are common, so when doing any lifting be sure to use proper body mechanics.

General Rules

- Never lift more than you can comfortably handle.

- Create a base of support by standing with your feet 8–12″ (shoulder width) apart with one foot a half step ahead of the other.

Proper foot position ▶

- DO NOT let your back do the heavy work—USE YOUR LEGS. (The back muscles are not your strongest muscles.)

- If the bed is low, put one foot on a footstool. This relieves pressure on your lower back.

- Consider using a support belt for your back.

Helpful Caregiver Advice for Moving a Person

These pointers are for the *caregiver* only. Be sure to see the following pages for the steps for a specific move or transfer.

◀ **1** • Tell the person what you are going to do.

• Before starting a move, count with the person, "1-2-3."

◀ **2** • To feel in control, get close to the person you are lifting.

• While lifting, keep your back in a neutral position (arched normally, not stiff), knees bent, weight balanced on both feet. Tighten your stomach and back muscles to maintain a correct support position.

• Use your arms to support the person.

• Again, *let your legs do the lifting.*

◀ **3** • Pivot (turn on one foot) instead of twisting your body.

• Breathe deeply.

• Keep your shoulders relaxed.

• When a lot of assistance is needed with transfers, tie a strong belt or a transfer belt around the person's waist and hold it as you complete the transfer.

Prevention of Back and Neck Injuries

To prevent injuries to yourself, get plenty of rest and maintain:

• good nutrition

• physical fitness

- good body mechanics

- a program for managing stress

Common Treatments for Caregiver Back Pain

If you *do* experience back pain:

- Apply a cold ice pack to the injured area for 10 minutes every hour (you can use a bag of frozen vegetables).

- Get short rest periods in a comfortable position.

- Stand with your feet about shoulder width apart and hands on hips, bend backwards. Do 3–5 repetitions several times a day.

- Take short, frequent walks on a level surface.

- Avoid sitting for long periods because sitting is one of the worst healing positions.

As the caregiver, you should seek training from a physical therapist to provide this type of care so as to reduce the risk of injury to yourself or the person in your care. The therapist will correct any mistakes you make and can take into account special problems. To determine the best procedure for you to use, the therapist will consider the physical condition of the person you care for and the furniture and room arrangements in the home.

Moving a Person

When you have to move someone—either in bed or out of bed—remember these tips:

- Plan the move and know what you can and cannot do.

- Let the person do as much work as he is capable of.

- Avoid letting the person put his arms around your neck or grab you.

- Use a transfer belt to balance and support the person.

- Place transfer surfaces (wheelchair and bed) close together.

- Check wheelchair position, **brakes locked**, armrests and footrests swung out of the way.

- Let the person look to the place where he is being transferred.

- If the person is able, place his hands on the bed or chair so he can assist in the movement. If the person has had a stroke or is afraid, have him clasp his hands close to his chest.

- Ask the person to *push* rather than *pull* on the bed rails, the chair, or you.

- Work at the person's level and speed and check for pain.

- Avoid sudden jerking motions.

- Never pull on the person's arms or shoulders.

- Correctly position the person. (This helps the body regain lost function and helps prevent additional function loss.)

- Have the person wear shoes with good treads or sturdy slippers.

 To encourage independence, let the person assist as he is able. It's okay for the person to stand up partly and sit back down.

Positioning a Person in Bed

1 ▶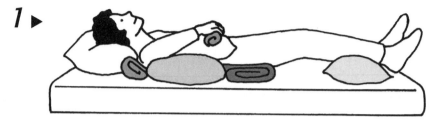

- Place a small pillow under the person's head, keeping his spine neutral.

- Place a small pillow lengthwise under the calf of the weak leg, let the heel hang off the end of the pillow to prevent pressure, and loosen the top sheet to avoid pressure on the toes.

2 ▶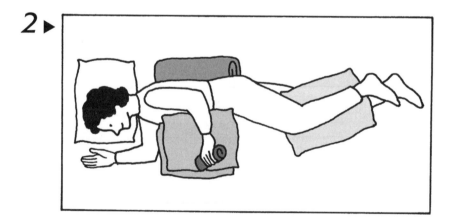

- Fold a bath towel under the hip of the person's weak side.

- Place the weak arm and elbow on a pillow higher than the heart.

Positioning a Person on His or Her Strong Side

1. Place a small pillow under the person's head.

2. Keep the person's head in alignment with the spine.

3. Place a rolled pillow at the back to prevent rolling.

4. Place a pillow in front to keep the arm the same height as the shoulder joint.

5. Place a medium pillow lengthwise between the knees, legs, and ankles. (The person's knees may be bent slightly.)

Positioning a Person on His or Her Weak Side

1. Use the same positioning as described above.

2. Change the person's position frequently because he may not be aware of pressure, pain, or skin irritation.

Moving a person in bed can injure the person in care or the caregiver if certain basic rules are not followed:

- Never grab or pull the person's arm or leg.

- If the medical condition allows, raise the foot of the bed slightly to prevent the person from sliding down.

- If moving him is difficult, get him out of bed and back in the wheelchair and start over by putting him in bed closer to the headboard.

Moving a Person Up in Bed

1. Tell the person what you are going to do.

2. Lower the head of the bed to a flat position and remove the pillow—never try to move the person "uphill."

3. If possible, raise the bed and **lock the wheels**.

4. Tell the person to bend his knees and brace his feet firmly against the mattress to help push.

5. Stand at the side of the bed and place one hand behind the person's back and the other underneath the buttocks.

6. Bend your knees and keep your back in a neutral position.

7. Count "1-2-3" and have the person push with his feet and pull with his hands toward the head of the bed.

8. Replace the pillow under his head.

Using Two People to Move an Unconscious Person

1
- Tell the person what you are going to do even if the person seems to be unconscious.
- Remove the pillow.
- If possible, raise the bed and **lock the wheels**.

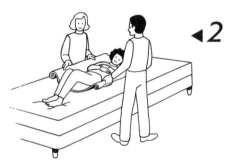

◀2
- Stand on either side of the bed.
- Face the head of the bed, with feet 8–12″ apart, knees bent, back in a neutral position.
- Roll the sides of the draw sheet up to the person's body.

◀3
- Grab the draw sheet with your palms up.
- Count "1-2-3" and then shift your body weight from the back to the front leg, keeping your arms and back in a locked position. Together, slide the person smoothly up the bed.
- Replace pillows under the person's head.
- Position the person comfortably.

A draw sheet—a sheet folded several times and positioned under the person to be moved in bed—prevents irritation to his skin. The sheet should be positioned from the shoulders to just below the knees.

Moving an Unconscious Person Alone

1. If possible, raise the whole bed and **lock the wheels**.

2. Remove the pillow.

3. Face the front of the bed, with feet 8–12″ apart, knees bent, back in a neutral position.

4. Roll the edge of the draw sheet and grab it.

5. Slide your arms under the draw sheet and the person's shoulders and back.

6. Count "1-2-3" and then shift your body weight from your back to front leg, keeping your arms and back in a locked position.

7. Slide the person to the top of the bed.

8. Replace the pillow.

9. Position the person comfortably.

PREVENTING BACK INJURIES
Having the person grab a trapeze to help with the move is easiest and safest for your back. (See p. 123.)

Moving the Person to One Side of the Bed on His or Her Back

1 • Place your feet 8–12″ apart, knees bent, back in a neutral position.

• Slide your arms under the person's back to her far shoulder blade. (Bend your knees and hips to lower yourself to the person's level.)

• Slide the person's shoulders toward you by rocking your weight to your back foot.

2 • Use the same procedure at the person's buttocks and feet.

• Always keep your knees bent and your back in a neutral position.

1 ▼   **2 ▼**

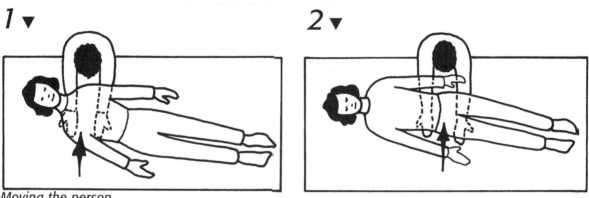

Moving the person

Rolling Technique

1. Move the person to one side of the bed as in the above procedure.

2. Bend the person's knees.

3. Hold the person at her hip and shoulder blade on the far side of the body.

4. Roll the person *toward* you to make sure she does not fall off the bed.

Raising the Person's Head and Shoulders

1. If possible, ask the person to lift her head and dig both elbows into the bed to support her body.

2. Face the head of the bed, feet 8–12″ apart, knees bent, back in neutral.

3. Help the person lift her shoulders by placing your hands and forearms under the pillow and her shoulder blades.

4. Use bent knees, back in neutral, and locked arms to assist the lift.

5. Adjust the pillow.

Helping a Person Sit Up

1. Tell the person what you are going to do.

2. Bend the person's knees.

3. Roll her on her side so she is facing you.

4. Reach one arm under her shoulder blade.

5. Place the other arm in back of her knees.

6. Position your feet 8–12″ apart with your center of gravity close to the bed and the person.

7. Keep your back in a neutral position.

8. Count "1-2-3" and shift your weight to your back leg.

9. Shift the person's legs over the edge of the bed while pulling her shoulders to a sitting position.

10. Remain in front of her until she is stabilized.

Transfers

Transferring a person in and out of bed is an important caregiver activity. It can be done fairly easily if these instructions are followed. Use the same procedure for all transfers so that a routine is set up.

Transfers Using a Mechanical Lift

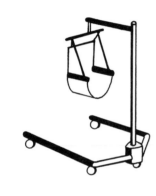

1. Tell the person what you are going to do.
2. Place the chair next to the bed with the back of the chair in line with the headboard of the bed. **Lock the wheels**.
3. Place a blanket or sheet over the chair.
4. Turn the person on one side toward the edge of the bed.
5. Fan-fold a sling and place it at the person's back.
6. Roll her to her other side, pull the sling out flat, and center it under her body.
7. Attach the sling to the mechanical lift with the hooks in place and facing out through the metal frame.
8. Fold the person's arms across her chest.
9. Using the crank, lift her out of bed.
10. Guide the legs. Lower her onto the chair.
12. Remove the hooks from the frame of the mechanical lift.
13. Leave the person in the chair with the sling under her, comfortably adjusted.
14. To get the person back in the bed, put the hooks facing out through the metal frame of the sling.
15. Raise the person using the crank.
16. Guide her legs. Lower her onto the bed.

17. Remove the hooks from the frame.

18. Remove the sling from under the person by turning her from side to side on the bed.

19. Properly position her with pillows. (📖 See p. 274.)

For lift instructions and precautions, refer to the *Positioning and Transfer Guide* that comes with your mechanical lift.

Helping a Person Stand

Help only as much as needed but guard the person from falling.

1. Have her sit on the edge of the chair or bed. Let her rest a moment if she feels lightheaded.

2. Instruct her to push off with her hands from the bed or chair armrests.

3. Position your knee between her knees.

4. Face her and support the weak knee against one or both of your knees as needed.

5. Put your arms around the person's waist or use a transfer belt.

6. Keep your back in a neutral position.

7. At the count of "1-2-3," instruct the person to stand up while pulling her toward you and pushing your knees into her knee if needed.

8. Once she is upright, have her keep her knee locked straight.

9. Support and balance her as needed.

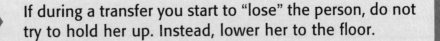

NOTE If during a transfer you start to "lose" the person, do not try to hold her up. Instead, lower her to the floor.

Helping a Person Sit

1. Reverse the process described in Helping a Person Stand.

2. Direct the person to feel for the chair or bed with the back of the legs.

3. Direct the person to reach back with both hands to the bed or chair armrests and slowly sit.

Transferring from Bed to Wheelchair with a Transfer Belt

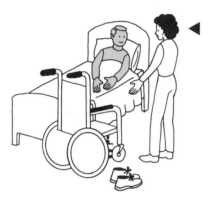

◄ **1** • Place the wheelchair at a 45° angle to the bed so that the person will be transferring to his stronger side.

• **Lock the wheels** of the chair and the bed.

• Tell the person what you are going to do.

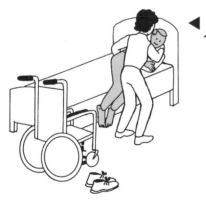

◄ **2** • Put on his shoes while he is still lying down if he is weak or unstable.

• Bring him to a sitting position with his legs over the edge of the bed.

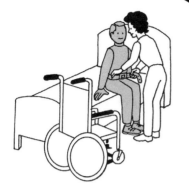

◀ **3** • Let him rest a moment if he feels lightheaded.

• Use a **transfer belt** for a person needing a lot of support.

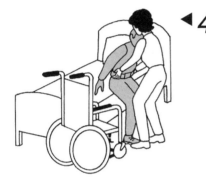

◀ **4** • Bring him to a standing position as described on page 281.

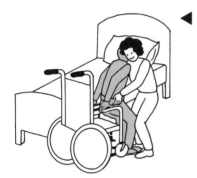

◀ **5** • Have him reach for the chair arm and pivot. A very fast pivot may frighten the person, or cause you to lose knee control and fall with a person who is totally dependent.

• Support him with your arms and knees as needed.

• Adjust him comfortably in the chair.

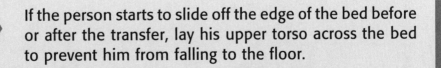

NOTE ▷ If the person starts to slide off the edge of the bed before or after the transfer, lay his upper torso across the bed to prevent him from falling to the floor.

Transferring from Wheelchair to Bed

1. Reverse the process described in Transfer from Bed to Wheelchair.

2. Place the chair at a 45° angle to the bed so the person is on his stronger side. **Lock the wheels**.

3. Get into a position to provide a good base of support; use good body mechanics.

4. Have the person stand, reach for the bed, and pivot.

5. Support and guide him as needed.

6. Adjust the person in bed with pillows.

Transferring from Bed to Wheelchair Without a Transfer Belt

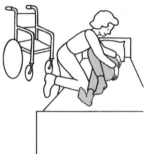

- Place the wheelchair at a 45° angle to the bed so that the person will be transferring to his stronger side.

- **Lock the wheels** of the chair (you can use a wheel block) and the wheels of the bed.

- Tell the person what you are going to do.

- Bring him to a sitting position with his legs over the edge of the bed following steps a, b, c, and d.

1a ▲

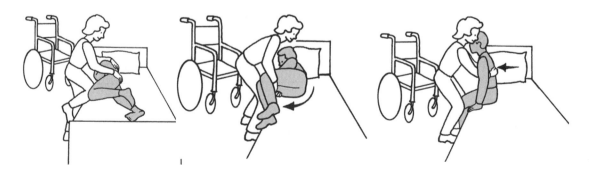

1b ▲   *1c* ▲   *1d* ▲

- Let him rest a moment if he feels lightheaded.
- Put his shoes on.

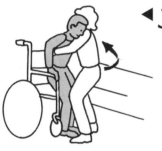

◀ **2** • Put your arms around his chest and clasp your hands behind his back.
- Support the leg that is farther from the wheelchair between your legs.

◀ **3** • Lean back, shift your leg, and lift.
- Pivot toward the chair.

◀ **4** • Bend your knees and let him bend toward you.
- Lower the person into the wheelchair.
- Adjust him comfortably in the chair.

NOTE ▶ As the person becomes stronger, you can provide less assistance. However, use the same body positioning to support the person's weaker side.

Transferring from Wheelchair to Bed with a Transfer Board

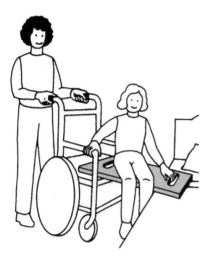

1. As much as possible, make the bed and the chair the same height.

2. Place the wheelchair at a 45° angle to the bed so that the person will be transferring to her stronger side.

3. **Lock the wheels** of the chair (you can use a wheel block) and the wheels of the bed.

4. Tell the person what you are going to do.

5. Remove the armrest nearest the bed.

6. Remove her feet from the footrests and swing the footrests out of the way.

7. Have the person lift her hip and place the board under the hip with the other end of the board on the bed.

8. MAKE SURE SHE DOESN'T PUT HER FINGERS UNDER THE BOARD.

9. Ask her to put her hands on the board with the hands close to her sides.

10. Ask her to lean slightly forward and to make a series of small pushes off the board by straightening her elbows and inching along the board toward the bed.

11. When she is on the bed, ask her to lean over onto her elbow and pull the transfer board out from under her bottom.

12. Adjust her comfortably in the bed.

Transferring from a Wheelchair to a Car

Be sure the car is parked on a level surface without cracks or potholes.

1 • Open the passenger door as far as possible.

• Move the left side of the wheelchair as close to the car seat as possible.

• **Lock the chair's wheels**.

• Move both footrests out of the way.

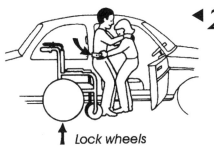

Lock wheels

◀*2* • Position yourself facing the person.

• Tell him what you are going to do.

• Bending your knees and hips, lower yourself to his level.

• By grasping the transfer belt around his waist help him stand while straightening your hips and knees.

• If his legs are weak, brace his knees with your knees.

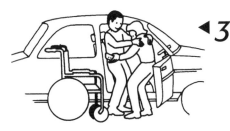

◀*3* • While he is standing, turn him so he can be eased down to sit on the car seat. GUIDE HIS HEAD so it is not bumped.

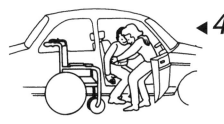

◀*4* • Lift his legs into the car by putting your hands under his knees.

• Move him to face the front.

• Put on his seat belt.

• Close door carefully.

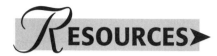

RESOURCES

American Academy of Orthopaedic Surgeons
6300 N. River Road
Rosemont, IL 60018
(800) 346-AAOS (800-346-2267)
www.aaos.org
Offers a free booklet Lift It Safe *on lifting procedures for home-based carergivers.*

If you don't have access to the Internet, ask your local library to help you locate a Web site.

Part Three: Additional Resources

Common Abbreviations

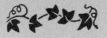

Acute MI – heart attack

ADA – Americans with Disabilities Act

ADL – activities of daily living

AFO – ankle-foot orthosis

ALF – assisted living facility

ASHD – arteriosclerotic heart disease

BC – blood culture

BID – 2 times per day (approximately 8 and 8 as medication times)

BP – blood pressure

BRP – bathroom privileges

BS – blood sugar

C&S – culture and sensitivity

CA – cancer/carcinoma

CABG – coronary artery bypass graft

CBC – complete blood count

CCU – coronary care unit

CHF – congestive heart failure

CNS – central nervous system

COPD – chronic obstructive pulmonary disease

CPR – cardiopulmonary resuscitation

CSF – cerebrospinal fluid

CVA – cerebral vascular accident

CVD – cerebral vascular disease

DM – diabetes mellitus

DME – durable medical equipment

DRG – diagnosis related group

Dx – diagnosis

ED – emergency department

EDSS – Expanded Disability Status Scale

EEG – electroencephalogram recording of the brain's electrical activity

EKG/ECG – electrocardiogram recording of the heart's electrical activity

EP – evoked potential

FBS – fasting blood sugar, or the amount of glucose in the blood when a person has not eaten for 12 hours

FX – fracture

GTT – glucose tolerance test to determine a person's ability to metabolize glucose

HC – home care

HHA – a home health agency providing home health services

HS – hour of sleep (medication time)

I&O – record of food and liquid taken in and waste eliminated

ICU – intensive care unit for special monitoring of the acutely ill

IV – intravenous line to drip fluids and blood products into the bloodstream

LOC – loss of consciousness

MCD – Medicaid

MCR – Medicare

MRI – magnetic resonance imaging

MS – multiple sclerosis

Neuro – neurologist

NPO – nothing by mouth

NSAID – nonsteroid anti-inflammatory drug.

OBS – organic brain syndrome, an injury or disorder that interferes with normal brain function

OR – operating room

OT – occupational therapy or occupational therapist

PO – by mouth

Psych – psychologist

PT – physical therapy or physical therapist

QID – 4 times per day (approximately 9–1–5–9 as medication times)

RBC – red blood count

RN – nurse

ROM – range of motion

RR – respiratory rate

RT – recreational therapy

Rx – prescription

SLP – speech-language pathologist

SNF – skilled nursing facility

SOB – shortness of breath

SS or SSA – Social Security or Social Security Administration

SSI/SSDI – supplemental security income or diability income

ST – Speech therapist or speech therapy

Sx – symptoms

TIA – transient ischemic attack

TID – 3 times per day (approximately 9–1–6 as medication times)

TPN – total parenteral nutrition

TPR – temperature, pulse, respiration

TX – treatment

U/A – urine analysis

VEP – visual evoked potential

VNS – visiting nurse service

WBC – white blood count

MS Specialists

Case Manager—a person (as a social worker or nurse) who assists in the planning, coordination, monitoring, and evaluation of medical services for a patient with emphasis on quality of care, continuity of services, and cost-effectiveness.

Chiropractor—A Doctor of Chiropractic specializes in a system of therapy with employs manipulation and specific adjustment of body structures (as the spinal column).

Counselors/mental health professionals—Help individuals and family members enhance problem-solving skills, grieve for losses, maintain self-esteem, handle changing relationships, learn to live with uncertainty, and find ways to be productive.

Family physician—Provides primary health care, including general health checkups, immunizations, and preventive care.

Massage Therapist—A professional specially trained in an assortment of techniques involving manipulation of the soft tissues of the body through pressure and movement.

MS nurse—Coordinates health care services. The nurse oversees initial and long-term management issues, teaches self-care, including taking of medications, and advocates with insurance companies and other agencies.

Neurologist—In addition to making the initial diagnosis, this professional prescribes treatments for MS and symptom management. The neurologist will refer you to other specialists as needed.

Neuro-ophthalmologist—a physician who specializes in the neurological study of the eye.

Neuropsychologist—Specializes in cognitive problems. The neuropsychologist can provide comprehensive neuropsychological testing and set up programs to compensate for cognitive issues identified in such evaluations.

Occupational therapist (OT)—Focuses mainly on skills that require upper body function. OTs are specialists in tools, techniques, or equipment to conserve energy and compensate (make up) for disabilities that affect activities of daily living.

Physiatrist—a physician specializing in physical medicine and rehabilitation, including the diagnosis and management of musculoskeletal injuries and pain syndromes, electrodiagnostic medicine (e.g., electromyography), and rehabilitation of severe impairments, including those caused by neurologic disease or injury.

Physical therapist (PT)—Focuses on exercise programs to reduce and prevent serious complications such as contractures (frozen joints) and osteoporosis, and to ease spasticity (spasms) and tremor (shaking). PTs (and occupational therapists) provide information on equipment and teach safe, effective ways to use these devices, including the best ways to transfer in and out of bed, a car, a shower, etc. PTs will help their clients create personal exercise programs for increasing stamina and preventing losses.

Radiologist—a physician specializing in the use of radiant energy for diagnostic and therapeutic purposes.

Social worker—Assesses social needs and links clients to community resources.

Speech/language pathologist (SLP)—Evaluates and treats speech and swallowing problems by training the person with MS, caregivers, and family members how to eat safely, prepare food that is easy to swallow, and manage feeding tubes if necessary. Some SLPs address cognitive issues as well.

Spiritual advisors/clergy—May support efforts to make sense of MS within a personal worldview. The choice of advisors and the sources of support are intensely personal matters but the need to pay attention to this aspect of life with MS cannot be overstated.

Other Specialists

Allergist/Immunologist
Disorders of the immune system

Anesthesiologist
Pain relief during and after surgery

Audiologist
Hearing disorders

Cardiologist
Conditions of the heart, lungs, and blood vessels

Chiropodist
Minor foot ailments such as corns and bunions

Colon and Rectal Surgeon
Diseases of the intestinal tract

Dentist
Teeth and gums

Dermatologist
Skin, hair, and nails

Endocrinologist
Hormonal problems including thyroid disorders

Forensic psychiatrist
Behavior assessment for legal purposes

Gastroenterologist
Digestive system, stomach, liver, bowels, and gallbladder

Geriatric psychiatrist
Emotional disorders of elderly persons

Geriatrician
Disorders common to elderly persons

Gynecologist
Female reproductive system

Hematologist
Diseases of the blood, spleen, and lymph glands

Internist
Primary care of common illnesses, both long term and emergency

Nephrologist
Kidney diseases and disorders

Neurologist
Brain and nervous system disorders

Oncologist
All cancers

Ophthalmologist
Care and surgery of the eyes

Optician
Fitting and making of eyeglasses and contact lenses

Optometrist
Basic eye care

Oral maxillofacial surgeon
Surgery involving the teeth, gums, and jaw

Orthopedist
Surgery involving joints, bones, and muscles

Orthotist
Nonmedical specialist in the measurement, sizing, and preparation of foot padding pieces

Osteopath (DO)
General medicine with emphasis on the promotion of health through the hands-on manipulation of the muscles, tendons, and joints.

Otolaryngologist
Head and neck surgeon

Pharmacist
Medications specialist; provider of physician and patient education

Podiatrist
Foot care

Psychiatrist (MD)
Emotional, mental, or addictive disorders

Psychologist (MA or PhD)
Assessment and care of emotional or mental disorders

Pulmonologist
Diseases of lungs and airways

Rheumatologist
Diseases of joints and connective tissue (arthritis)

Urologist
Urinary system and the male reproductive system

International MS and Caregiver Organizations

Multiple Sclerosis Australia
www.msaustralia.org.au
(61) 02 9646 0600
Multiple Sclerosis Australia strives for a world without multiple sclerosis through quality research, and for service excellence for people with multiple sclerosis and their caregivers.

Multiple Sclerosis International Federation
www.msif.org
The Federation seeks to work in worldwide partnership with member societies and the international scientific community to eliminate multiple sclerosis and its consequences, and to speak out globally on behalf of those affected by multiple sclerosis. The Federation maintains a database of MS Societies throughout the world.

Multiple Sclerosis Society of Canada
www.mssociety.ca
(416) 922-6065
The mission of the Multiple Sclerosis Society of Canada is "To be a leader in finding a cure for multiple sclerosis and enabling people affected by MS to enhance their quality of life." Our two major programs provide hope for the future through the support of MS research into the cause, treatment, and cure of the disease and hope for today through our many services that assist people with MS and their families.

Multiple Sclerosis Society of Great Britain and Northern Ireland

www.mssociety.org.uk
(44) 020 8438 0700
The Society's aims and objectives are:

- *To support and relieve people affected by MS*

- *To encourage people affected by MS to attain their full potential as members of society by improving their lives.*

- *To promote research into MS and allied conditions and to publish results.*

Multiple Sclerosis Society of Ireland Ltd.

www.ms-society.ie
353 1 678 1601
MS Helpline 1850 233 233
The mission of MS Ireland is to enable and empower people with MS to live the life of their choosing to their fullest potential.

National Multiple Sclerosis Society

www.nationalmssociety.org
(800) FIGHT-MS (800-344-4867)
The mission of the National Multiple Sclerosis Society is to end the devastating effects of MS. Founded in 1946, the National Multiple Sclerosis Society supports more MS research, offers more services for people with MS, provides more professional education programs, and furthers more MS advocacy efforts than any other MS organization in the world. Studies show that early and ongoing treatment with an FDA-approved therapy can reduce future disease activity and improve quality of life for many people with multiple sclerosis. Talk to your health care professional and contact the National Multiple Sclerosis Society at www.nationalms-society.org or (800) FIGHT-MS to learn about ways to help manage multiple sclerosis and about current research that may one day reveal a cure.

International Caregiver Organizations

AUSTRALIA

Carers Australia
www.carersaustralia.com.au
(800) 242-636
Carers Australia represents the needs and interests of caregivers at the national level by

- *Advocating for carers' needs and interests in the public arena*

- *Influencing government and stakeholder policies and programs at the national level through conducting research and pilot projects, giving presentations, and participating in a wide range of inquiries, reviews, and policy forums*

- *Networking and forming strategic partnerships with other organizations to achieve positive outcomes for carers*

- *Providing carers with information and education resources, undertaking community activities to raise awareness, and coordinating and facilitating joint work between the state and territory organizations on matters of national significance*

CANADA

Canadian Caregiver Coalition
www.ccc-ccan.ca
The Canadian Caregivers Coalition helps identify and respond to the needs of caregivers in Canada.

Caregiver Network, Inc.
www.caregiver.on.ca/
(416) 323-1090
Based in Toronto, Canada, CNI's goal is to be a national single-information source to make your life as a caregiver easier.

UNITED KINGDOM

Carers UK
www.carersuk.org
Carers UK is the leading campaigning, policy, and information organization for carers. We are a membership organization, led and set up by carers in 1965 to have a voice and to win the recognition and support that carers deserve.

UNITED STATES

FamilyCare *America*, Inc.
1004 N. Thompson St., Suite 205
Richmond, VA 23230
(804) 342-2200
www.FamilyCareAmerica.com
FamilyCare America is dedicated to improving the lives of caregivers of the elderly, disabled, and chronically ill by creating a highly accessible resource where caregivers can:

- *better learn the process of caregiving*

- *receive help in managing their fears and concerns*

- *obtain resources for help with all aspects of caregiving*

National Alliance for Caregiving
4720 Montgomery Lane, 5th Floor
Bethesda, MD 20814
www.caregiving.org
The Alliance is a non-profit coalition of national organizations focusing on issues of family caregiving.

National Family Caregivers Association
10400 Connecticut Avenue, Suite 500
Kensington, MD 20895
(800) 896-3650
The Association supports, empowers, educates, and speaks up for the more than 50 million Americans who care for a chronically ill, aged, or disabled person.

National Quality Caregiving Coalition (NQCC)
750 First Street, NE
Washington, DC 20002-4242
(202) 336-5606
www.nqcc-rci.org
The NQCC is a coalition of national associations, groups, and individuals with interests in and active agendas that promote caregiving across all ages and disabilities throughout the lifespan.

Well Spouse Association
63 West Main Street—Suite H
Freehold, NJ 07728
(800) 838-0879
www.wellspouse.org
Well Spouse is a national, not-for-profit membership organization that gives support to wives, husbands, and partners of the chronically ill and/or disabled.

Glossary

A

Activities of daily living (ADL): personal hygiene, bathing, dressing, grooming, toileting, feeding, and transferring

Acute: state of illness that comes on suddenly and may be of short duration

Adult day care: supervised centers where older or disabled adults can be with others

Advance directive: a legal document that states a person's health care preferences in writing while that person is competent and able to make such decisions

Affected release: also called pseudo-bulbar affect or pathological laughing and weeping; a condition in which episodes of laughing and/or crying occur with no apparent precipitating event. The person's actual mood may be unrelated to the emotion being expressed. This condition is thought to be caused by lesions in the limbic system, a group of brain structures involved in emotional feeling and expression.

Ambulatory: able to walk with little or no assistance

Analgesics: medications used to relieve pain

Antibiotics: a group of drugs used to combat infection

Anxiety: a state of discomfort, dread, and foreboding with physical symptoms such as rapid breathing and heart rate, tension, jitters, and muscle aches

Aromatherapy: use of essential oils of various plants to treat symptoms of diseases, improve sleep, and reduce stress by inducing relaxation

Artificial life-support systems: the use of respirators, tube feeding, intravenous (IV) feeding, and other means to replace natural and vital functions, such as breathing, eating, and drinking

*For a more complete glossary of MS terms, visit the National Multiple Sclerosis Society's Web site at www.nationalmssociety.org/glossary

Assessment: the process of studying and analyzing a person's condition

Assisted living: residential housing offering independence, choice of services, and assistance with activities of daily living, including meals and housekeeping

Assistive devices: any tools that are designed, fabricated, and/or adapted to assist a person in performing a particular task, e.g., cane, walker, shower chair

Assistive technology: a term used to describe all of the tools, products, and devices, from the simplest to the most complex, that can make a particular function easier or possible to perform

Atrophy: the wasting away of muscles or brain tissue

B

Bedpan: a container into which a person urinates and defecates while in bed

Blood pressure: the pressure of the blood on the walls of the blood vessels and arteries

Body language: gestures that serve as a form of communication

Body mechanics: proper use and positioning of the body to do work and avoid strain and injury

C

Calorie: the measure of the energy the body gets from various foods

Catheter: a rubber tube for collecting urine from a person who has become incontinent

Chronic: a state or condition that lasts 6 months or longer

Cognition: high-level functions carried out by the human brain, including comprehension and use of speech, visual perception and construction, calculation ability, attention (information processing), memory, and executive functions such as planning, problem-solving, and self-monitoring

Cognitive rehabilitation: techniques designed to improve the functioning of individuals whose cognition is impaired because of physical trauma or disease

Congregate living: a type of independent living in which people can live in their own apartments but have meals, laundry, transportation, and housekeeping services available

Conservator: a person given the power to take over and protect the interests of one who is incompetent

Constipation: difficulty having bowel movements

Contracture: shortening or tightening of the tissue around a joint so that the person loses the ability to move easily

D

Decubitus ulcer: pressure sore; bedsore

Defibrillator: a device that uses and electrical current to restore or regulate a stopped or disorganized heartbeat

Dehydration: loss of normal body fluid, sometimes caused by vomiting and severe diarrhea

Depression: a psychiatric condition that can be moderate or severe and cause feelings of sadness and emptiness

Diuretics: drugs that help the body get rid of fluids

Draw sheet: a sheet folded widthwise to position under someone in bed to keep the linen clean and aid in transfers

Durable power of attorney: a legal document that authorizes another to act as one's agent and is "durable" because it remains in effect in case the person becomes disabled or mentally incompetent

Durable power of attorney for health care decisions: a legal document that lets a person name someone else to make health care decisions after the person has become disabled or mentally incompetent and is unable to make those decisions

Dysarthria: poorly articulated speech resulting from dysfunction of the muscles controlling speech, usually caused by damage to the central nervous system or a peripheral motor nerve; the content and meaning of the spoken words remain normal

Dysphagia: difficulty swallowing

Dysphonia: disorders of voice quality (including poor pitch control, hoarseness, breathiness, and hypernasality) caused by spasticity, weakness, and incoordination of muscles in the mouth and throat

E

Edema: an abnormal swelling in legs, ankles, hands, or abdomen that occurs because the body is retaining fluids

Estate planning: a process of planning for the present and future use of a person's assets

Evoked potentials (EPs): EPs are recordings of the nervous system's electrical response to the stimulation of specific sensory pathways (e.g., visual, auditory, general sensory)

Expanded Disability Status Scale (EDSS): a part of the Minimal Record of Disability that summarizes the neurologic examination and provides a measure of overall disability

➶ F

Foster care: a care arrangement in which a person lives in a private home with a primary caregiver and 4 or 5 other people

Foot drop: a condition of weakness in the muscles of the foot and ankle, caused by poor nerve conduction, which interferes with a person's ability to flex the ankle and walk with a normal heel–toe pattern; the toes touch the ground before the heel, causing the person to trip or lose balance

➶ G

Guardian: the one who is designated to have protective care of another person or of that person's property

➶ H

Heimlich maneuver: a method for clearing the airway of a choking person

Hemorrhage: excessive bleeding

Hospice: a program that allows a dying person to remain at home while receiving professionally supervised care

➶ I

Immune system: a complex network of glands, tissues, circulating cells, and processes that protect the body by identifying abnormal or foreign substances and neutralizing them

Impaction: inability to pass gas or have bowel movements

Incontinence: involuntary discharge of urine or feces

Intravenous (IV): the delivery of fluids, medications, or nutrients into a vein

Involved: a term used to describe the side of the body most affected by a disease, operation, or medical condition

❧ L

L-Hermitte's sign: an abnormal sensation of electricity or "pins and needles" going down the spine into the arms and legs that occurs when the neck is bent forward so that the chin touches the chest

Laxative: a substance taken to increase bowel movements and prevent constipation

❧ M

Mechanical lift: a machine used to lift a person from one place to another (Hoyer lift)

MedicAlert®: a bracelet identification system that is linked to a 24-hour service that provides full information in the case of an emergency

Medicaid: a public health program that uses state and federal funds to pay certain medical and hospital expenses of those having low income or no income, with benefits that vary from state to state

Medicare: the federal health insurance program for people 65 or older and for certain people under 65 who are disabled

❧ N

Nutrition: supplying the body with the key nutrients it needs for proper body function

Nystagmus: rapid, involuntary movements of the eyes in the horizontal or, occasionally, the vertical direction

❧ O

Occupational therapy: therapy that focuses on the activities of daily living such as personal hygiene, bathing, dressing, grooming, toileting, and feeding

Ombudsman: a person who helps residents of a retirement or health care facility with such problems as quality of care, food, finances, medical care, residents rights, and other concerns; these services are confidential and free

Optic neuritis: inflammation or demyelination of the optic (visual) nerve with transient or permanent impairment of vision and occasionally pain

Oral hygiene: the process of keeping the mouth clean

Oscillopsia: continuous, involuntary, and chaotic eye movements that result in a visual disturbance in which objects appear to be jumping or bouncing

৵ P

Paralysis: loss or impairment of voluntary movement of a group of muscles

Paraparesis: a weakness, but not total paralysis, of the lower extremities (legs)

Paresthesia: a spontaneously occurring sensation of burning, prickling, tingling, or creeping on the skin that may or may not be associated with any physical findings on neurologic examination

Pathogen: a disease-causing microorganism

Physical therapy: the process of relearning walking, balancing, and transfers

Pocketing: getting food caught between the cheek and the gum on the paralyzed side of face

Posey: a vest-like restraint used to keep a person from getting out of bed

Positioning: placing a person in a position that allows functional activity and minimizes the danger of faulty posture that could cause pressure sores, impaired breathing, and shrinking of muscles and tendons

Power of attorney for health care: a document for providing another person with the authority to make health care decisions

Pressure sore: breakdown of the skin caused by prolonged pressure in one spot; a bed sore; decubitus ulcer

Prone: position of the body lying down

Pseudo-exacerbation: a temporary aggravation of disease symptoms, resulting from an elevation in body temperature or other stressor (e.g., an infection, severe fatigue, constipation) that disappears once the stressor is removed. A pseudo-exacerbation involves symptom flare-up rather than new disease activity or progression

৵ Q

Quadriplegia: paralysis of both the upper and lower parts of the body from the neck down

৵ R

Range of motion (ROM): the extent of possible passive (movement by another person) movement in a joint

Rehabilitation: after a disabling injury or disease, restoration of a person's maximum physical, mental, vocational, social, and spiritual potential

Representative payee: a person who receives Social Security benefits paid on someone else's behalf

Respite care: short-term care that allows a primary caregiver time off from his or her responsibilities

୬ର S

Sedatives: medications used to calm a person

Shock: a state of collapse resulting from reduced blood volume and blood pressure caused by burns, severe injury, pain, or an emotional blow

Spasticity: feelings of stiffness and a wide range of involuntary muscle spasms (sustained muscle contractions or sudden movements)

Speech therapy: the treatment of disorders of communication, including expressive language, writing, and reading and communication required for activities of daily living

Supine: lying on one's back

Support groups: groups of people who get together to share common experiences and help one another cope

Symptom: sign of a disease or disorder

୬ର T

Tracheotomy: surgical procedure to make an opening in a person's windpipe to aid in breathing

Tranquilizers: a class of drugs used to calm a person and control certain emotional disturbances

Transfer: movements from one position to another, for example, from bed to chair, wheelchair to car, etc.

Transfer belt: a device placed around the waist of a disabled person and used to secure the person while walking; a gait belt

Transfer board (sliding board): polished wooden or plastic board used to slide a person when moving from one place to another, for example, bed to wheelchair or commode

Trapeze: a metal bar suspended over a bed to help a person raise up or move

Trigeminal neuralgia: lightning-like, acute pain in the face caused by demyelination of nerve fibers at the site where the sensory (trigeminal) nerve root for that part of the face enters the brainstem

➤ U

Urinal: a container used by a bedridden male for urinating

Urinalysis: a laboratory test of urine

➤ V

Vital signs: life signs such as blood pressure, breathing, pulse, and temperature

Void: to urinate; pass water

➤ W

Will: a legal document that states how to dispose of a person's property after death according to that person's wishes

Index